They Took My Wife's Breast

THEY
TOOK
MY
WIFE'S
Breast

KEN OLIVE

NEW YORK

LONDON • NASHVILLE • MELBOURNE • VANCOUVER

They Took My Wife's Breast

Published in New York, New York, by Morgan James Publishing. Morgan James is a trademark of Morgan James, LLC. www.MorganJamesPublishing.com

The Morgan James Speakers Group can bring authors to your live event. For more information or to book an event visit The Morgan James Speakers Group at www.TheMorganJamesSpeakersGroup.com.

Scripture quotations are from the Holy Bible, New International Version®, NIV®. Copyright © 1973, 1978, 1984, 2011 by Biblica, Inc. ™ Used by permission of Zondervan. All rights reserved worldwide. www.zondervan.com. The "NIV" and "New International Version" are trademarks registered in the United States Patent and Trademark Office by Biblica, Inc. ™>>

ISBN 9781683508328 paperback
ISBN 9781683508342 case laminate
ISBN 9781683508335 eBook
Library of Congress Control Number: 2017917167

Cover and Interior Design by:
Chris Treccani
www.3dogcreative.net

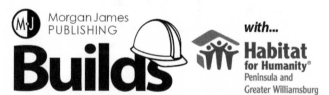

In an effort to support local communities, raise awareness and funds, Morgan James Publishing donates a percentage of all book sales for the life of each book to Habitat for Humanity Peninsula and Greater Williamsburg.

Get involved today! Visit
www.MorganJamesBuilds.com

For my Phyllis

Contents

Chapter 1

THE LUMP

Phyllis had found another lump in her left breast. She didn't even bother to tell me, her husband. She'd found other cysts and simply had them drained in the past, so she didn't worry about it.

Just before her scheduled annual routine mammogram, she mentioned the lump to me. I did as she asked and checked it out. It was very hard, almost like a small rock. I assured her it was probably just another cyst, and she agreed. She didn't seem fretful about it, and I wasn't either.

She kept her appointment with her gynecologist, Dr. Stephen Allen, on Friday, July 11, 2014, and told him about the lump. He examined her, then sent her in to the mammogram technician. There her breasts were flattened out between the two horizontal panels on the x-ray machine. Just thinking about it makes me cringe. I had always figured the woman simply walked up to the x-ray machine and put her chest against the cold panel and then the technician snapped the picture from the inside of their closet made of lead. I was wrong.

That evening Phyllis and I were relaxing at home after work when I asked her how the exam went. She said everything went smoothly. She wouldn't get the results until Monday. I didn't think about it anymore.

Phyllis worked all weekend and then headed to Birmingham, Alabama, from our home in Tuscaloosa, Alabama, in her little black BMW. Our daughter Caroline and her family were there for the 2014 Southeastern Conference Media Days. I didn't get to join her on her trip because I had not worked all weekend like her. Phyllis is a Realtor with RE/MAX Premiere Group in Tuscaloosa where I'm the Qualifying Broker and owner of the company. She hit the road while I went into the office.

As Phyllis navigated the seemingly endless road construction on Interstate 59 between Tuscaloosa and Birmingham, her phone alerted her that a call was coming in from Dr. Allen's office. She was nervous when she answered the call, not knowing what to expect. Dr. Allen simply said, "It looks suspicious. We need to get a biopsy."

I was crunching numbers in my office when Phyllis called and relayed what Dr. Allen had said. I immediately began to sharpen my focus—the numbers in front of me blurred. I asked Phyllis if she was expecting this, and she admitted that something about this lump seemed different to her. I tried to assure her that the biopsy results would be fine. I reminded her how healthy she was and how well she took care of herself. She agreed, and we changed the subject to her plans with Caroline in Birmingham. I was rambling, talking about nothing really, and avoiding the topic on both of our minds. She ended the call, heading on to Birmingham and I leaned back in the chair at my desk, thinking about her biopsy.

Phyllis arrived at The Hyatt Wynfrey Hotel in Birmingham shaken but forcing a smile for Caroline and our granddaughters, Olivia and Marlys. SEC Media Days is a big deal if you're a college football fan—and we all tend to be big fans in Alabama. All the head coaches and a few players from the SEC were staying there at the Hyatt Wynfrey Hotel, taking interviews with news outlets from across the region. Caroline's husband A.J. Mockler worked with the SEC Network as an audio specialist, and he'd invited Caroline and the girls along to enjoy the fun during his breaks. Olivia was five years old at the time and Marlys was three.

Phyllis met them at the Riverchase Galleria food court, which is in the same mall at the hotel. As Phyllis walked up, the granddaughters were playing at the carousel at the food court. Caroline greeted her and noticed right away that something was off. She asked if something was wrong at the office. When Phyllis shared her serious news from Dr. Allen, raw emotion overcame them both. After shedding a few tears, they spotted the girls heading their way. "Gigi!" they called as they raced to see her. Phyllis steeled herself and greeted them warmly. It's always been about the children with Phyllis.

Phyllis and Caroline made themselves have a nice time and got a few pictures of everyone on the set of SEC Nation, pretending to be one of the famous announcers on the show. All the girls looked better than Paul Finebaum, one of the show's hosts, sitting there on the set!

After the day's activities wound down and dinner was over, they crashed in the hotel room with double beds. Marlys and Olivia had to sleep with their Gigi, and Caroline and A.J. were together in the other bed—earplugs were available for anyone that needed

Phyllis was restless that night with her mind racing and playing out all the different scenarios that could play out after the biopsy.

them to drown out the snoring. No need to get into who needed them and who did not!

Phyllis was restless that night with her mind racing and playing out all the different scenarios that could play out after the biopsy. She was wide awake when morning finally came, lying in the bed waiting for the others to stir. Quietly, Caroline crawled into bed with Phyllis and the girls. She began praying for Phyllis out loud—praying for God's healing and strength, claiming victory the way only a prayer warrior can. My baby girl was trying to be strong for her mother, telling her that everything would be all right because she would continue to pray. Suddenly her chin started quivering, and she began to cry. Soon, it was mother comforting daughter, with Phyllis telling Caroline everything was going to be all right. That was the moment Phyllis realized even if she had breast cancer, she still had to be strong for her family. She did not waiver from that commitment.

Dr. Allen had recommended Phyllis to one surgeon who wanted to schedule her biopsy thirty days later. She politely insisted the biopsy be scheduled sooner. She didn't want to delay it thirty days without knowing what the prognosis would be. I thought, "That's my wife! *Let's get on with it!*" Dr. Allen recommended Dr. Andy Harrell who promptly put her on the schedule for that Wednesday.

So, Phyllis cut her SEC Media Days trip short for the biopsy. I drove her to the Tuscaloosa Surgical Center where the biopsy would be performed. We were familiar with the place, having been there a few times over the years for minor procedures with family and friends. It was a modern building made of stucco and glass on McFarland Boulevard, just three minutes from our home.

We walked into the Surgical Center at 7:30 a.m., and the waiting room was already full. As soon as we got there, Phyllis started telling me to leave and go on to the office, insisting when it was over I could come back and pick her up. I obliged, knowing she was her father's daughter and nothing should get in the way of work. After a short wait and making sure she was situated with the nurses, I went on to the office.

Concentrating at my office proved impossible, so I returned to the Surgical Center by midmorning. One of the nurses took me through the metal doors and down a corridor wide enough for two rolling beds to pass each other. Cubicles were on either side of the hallway and were separated with tall curtains hanging from metal rings. As I took in my surroundings I realized this wasn't a place a healthy person longed to be. Most of the people here were just like me and Phyllis and were not here by choice. I was praying our news would be good and even said a little prayer for everyone else there that day.

Most of the morning's patients were behind the curtains, but Phyllis had scored a private room with a glass front wall that allowed the nurses to keep an eye on her. Our friend Karen Smelley was her nurse, and as she slid the glass door back, Phyllis looked up and smiled at me. She was still groggy from the anesthesia, but through the fog, her top lip would occasionally quiver—a tell I had seen many times before that indicated she was nervous or about to cry. I kept a stiff upper lip for the both of us.

She was being cared for like a celebrity, but they wouldn't discharge her until her body cleared itself of the drugs. Looking back, I think they were all pretty sure it was breast cancer. As many times as those doctors and nurses had performed similar biopsies, they must have had a sense for whether it's good or bad. After a couple of hours, she was good to go. I collected her personal items and did as the nurse instructed and went to get our car to pull it around front under the awning. When I drove up, she was impatiently waiting in the wheel chair, ready to get back to work.

I left the Surgical Center troubled, fearing the worst but keeping it to myself. Now we had to wait for the verdict, and the next day was Phyllis' birthday.

Chapter 2

HAPPY BIRTHDAY, PHYLLIS!

The next day, with the results still pending from the biopsy, Phyllis, our son, Russell, Caroline, A.J., and our granddaughters, Olivia and little Marlys all loaded up and went to dinner at Firebirds Wood Fired Grill to celebrate Phyllis' fifty-seventh birthday. Firebirds serves great steaks and seafood, and it was Phyllis' birthday dinner choice. Everybody was trying hard to be festive, but with the news Phyllis had shared, we all were thinking to ourselves that bad news might be coming.

Phyllis decided she wanted champagne, and we let her have at it! Not that it was left up to us!

I can't remember much of our conversations that evening, but I do remember that throughout dinner I was wondering how involved the lumps would be. At this point I had no idea and was imagining the worst. Russell was quiet, worried about his mother, and Caroline and Phyllis were carrying the conversation while everyone else was busy tending to Marlys and Olivia. I think those granddaughters bumped her biopsy incision a hundred times that night. I wasn't very much fun that evening, I'm sure.

The meal was excellent, and we did have a big laugh about dessert. It was silly, and maybe we were searching for anything to laugh at. At the time, salted caramel was becoming a popular flavor, and the cute, tattooed waitress informed us that one of the desserts had salted caramel in it. Phyllis said, "OH! Salty caramel!" She could not wait until the "salty caramel" dessert arrived and kept mentioning it until it arrived. We were ALL happy when the dessert came out! You had to be there to get it. We still make jokes about salty caramel.

> *Phyllis later admitted she was thinking, "If I'm going to die, I'm going to die enjoying champagne and eating dessert!"*

Phyllis later admitted she was thinking, "If I'm going to die, I'm going to die enjoying champagne and eating dessert!" I feigned courage and told her everything was going to be all right.

When the party was over, Russell and I headed back to Tuscaloosa, and Phyllis left with Caroline and her crew for one more night at The Hyatt Wynfrey Hotel. It was a nice little trip for Phyllis, and it gave her a distraction from reality. But as Vivian Leigh tearfully said in *Gone with the Wind,* "Tomorrow is another day."

Chapter 3

BIOPSY RESULTS

The afternoon of July 18, 2014, Phyllis and I were in our kitchen when she got the call from Dr. Harrell. She was on her way to show a $500,000 condo on the University of Alabama campus, and I happened to be home at the time, which was odd for me. I believe God had a hand in it. I was leaning against the kitchen island listening in on the telephone call, and she was leaning against the kitchen counter by the door. When the call ended, she didn't collapse or get in a fetal position, but her big brown eyes welled up with tears. She simply said, "It's breast cancer, Ken". Dr. Harrell had told her she had Ductal Carcinoma in Situ (DCIS). I wrapped her up in a hug and said, "We'll deal with it." We had dealt with many obstacles before throughout our marriage, and we would deal with this breast cancer together too.

All I could think was: I don't want her to die. This family needs her. She's been my friend and buddy since high school. My wife and lover for 39 years. She can't have cancer! Phyllis later told me her

We had dealt with many obstacles before throughout our marriage, and we would deal with this breast cancer together too.

initial thought was: Am I going to die? That was followed with: Will I lose my breasts? What will Ken think of me? Can I survive all the treatments? Will I see my granddaughters grow up?

I must admit it was not a moment of great faith for me.

Chapter 4

GROWING UP

P hyllis and I both grew up in the country and were taught to include "Ma'am" or "Sir" in front of "yes" or "no." We were both blessed with loving parents. Neither of us would change our roots one iota. I was a preacher's kid with an older brother and sister, and I did my best to live up to what people usually say about preacher's kids. Phyllis was the middle child of five with one sister, three brothers, a kind-hearted mother named Doris, and an insanely hard-working father named Johnny.

Growing up in Samantha, Alabama, home of the Northside High School Rams, Phyllis and I lived about two miles apart. I had a simple life. Playing outdoors all day until my mother, JoAnn, called for me and made me come inside because it was "getting dark." With my dad, Jim, being a minister, we went to church every time the doors were open— the first ones there, last ones to leave—every Sunday morning, Sunday night, and Wednesday night prayer meeting. Oh yeah, we sometimes had revivals and, the thing I disliked the most, all-day singings. I have to admit that growing up I was not a fan of church. Had it not been for friends like Darrell Sullivan, I probably would not have survived. Darrell and I spent countless hours throwing footballs, baseballs, or shooting basketball after church and on Sunday afternoons. We played whatever was in season and we lived for sports, especially Alabama football and basketball. Darrell became a minister and I did not. I've said in the past that I had enough church as a child to last me a lifetime, though I say it with a smile.

While I was serving my sentence at church, Phyllis was riding motorcycles and horses, daydreaming of flying away on one of the jets overhead to Europe to be with Cary Grant and ride in his convertible like Grace Kelly. All was not playing and daydreaming for her, though. Her daddy always had chores for those kids to do. But she always had someone to play with. With five kids that usually had friends over, there was always enough for a friendly game of kickball or intense foot races. Phyllis claims she could outrun her slightly older brother, Ricky, and this caused no small discord between the two at the time. Sibling rivalry at its best!

As the baby of my family (my mother called me her baby until the day she died), I didn't have the sibling rivalries. My older brother and sister always told anyone who would listen that I was in a class by myself. I'm not sure if they were complimenting me or not.

My first memory of Phyllis was when I was in grammar school at Gorgas Elementary. She got on Mr. Olan Oswalt's school bus, and I thought she was skinny but pretty. She was a grade ahead of me, and at that point she was only an observation to me. Phyllis was a close friend with my cousin, Debbie Hudson, and they had their own little gang that included Celia Jo Gilliam and Linda Kuykendall. I thought them to be silly girls who believed they were better than me, and Debbie called me a heathen. Debbie was a do-gooder and I didn't relate to that.

The first time I really noticed Phyllis was in my high school sophomore year. I had been asked by my older brother Ronnie and his friend Randy to maybe set them up with her because they thought she was pretty. They knew I was friends with most everyone at school and that I wasn't afraid to talk to girls. A few days later I was walking down the school hallway, and I looked through the door of our favorite English Literature teacher Mrs. Josephine Gustafson's class.

There sat Phyllis on the front row in a miniskirt, long legs crossed and swinging her foot.

There sat Phyllis on the front row in a miniskirt, long legs crossed and swinging her foot. She smiled as I walked by. It wasn't a pleased-to-make-your-acquaintance smile. It was a Joey-from-*Friends* "How you doin?" smile. With a testosterone-driven confidence, I stepped back a few steps for another look—and to make sure she saw me smile back. From that moment on, Ronnie and Randy would receive no further help from me. Sorry, bro, I wanted to get to know her better myself. I thought she was beautiful and she thought I was cute, and when you are teenagers . . . well, that's enough. I pray dementia never takes that memory from me.

So, since I was fifteen years of age and even before that really, Phyllis has been a part of my life. She was my Homecoming Queen and as her King, I increased my status greatly among my male friends. She cheered me on while I played basketball for the Rams, and I watched her play volleyball and softball. We were together constantly and shared many good memories.

Like the time she took me to get my driver's license on my sixteenth birthday. That's right! Unlike some kids today, my friends and I counted the days until we became licensed to drive. Most of us went on our birthday to the Tuscaloosa County Courthouse to prove to the world that we could parallel park and get our license. I still can't believe that as a junior, she even considered dating a sophomore, not old enough for a driver's license. I guess that proves how small the dating pool was at Northside High School!

Anyhow, on September 24, 1974, Phyllis drove me to the Courthouse to get my driver's license. We were in my old family car—a four-door, green with a black, vinyl roof, Toyota Corona, which had unofficially become my car. I parallel parked perfectly for State Trooper Estes, passed the test, and officially became a licensed driver and *the* driver for us. I think we celebrated by getting a pizza at Pizza Hut. There have only been a few times since then that Phyllis has driven us, and that suits us both.

With a girlfriend and a car, I now needed more income. Finding odd jobs for a country boy willing to work wasn't that hard, and I was willing. My jobs consisted of hauling hay and cutting grass, but I wanted more work. Phyllis' dad Johnny offered to let me work with him on Saturdays. He was a logger (lumberjack to Northerners) that was not known for his patience, but while training me those Saturdays, he showed me more patience than I deserved. He was testing me and I knew it, but he taught me what real work was and I was already pretty tough.

The Saturday work evolved into a summer job where I earned enough money to take Johnny's daughter on dates and, eventually, to buy an engagement ring. I asked Phyllis to marry me the Christmas of my high school senior year. She said yes! On June 18, 1976, one month after I graduated, we were married by my father at the little country church where he pastored. I was seventeen and she was eighteen. We thought we knew everything. I was happy and knew I had married way up!

We set about building a life together by both working hard and saving enough money to build a home after two years of marriage. A few years later, we started a family. First came our big baby boy, Russell, and a couple of years later my beautiful baby girl, Caroline. Phyllis was in charge of most of their raising while they were young children, but when they became teenagers, I turned into the parent who was in charge. I was the dad that couldn't go to sleep until they came home, and Phyllis knew that our teenagers were well aware their Daddy was waiting up for them. She peacefully slept knowing I would handle them if they deviated from their curfew. We sent them to college, and now they are each successful in their own right with beautiful families of their own.

It wasn't all Pleasantville, however. We suffered through some financial tough times. We lost both my parents and Phyllis' father, and those were hard losses. But we are still here together as a team. We finish each other's sentences and help the other remember a forgotten name, and she allows me control of the remote. I taught her how to handle a bully, and she taught me to hold my temper. I buy Blue Bell Ice Cream, and she buys yogurt.

So, *of course* we would deal with breast cancer together! I never considered anything else. My only question was how could I help Phyllis fight? I have felt helpless few times in my life, but the day I discovered she had breast cancer is at the top of the list. I couldn't protect her from breast cancer, and I couldn't make it all better like some little boo-boo. I couldn't go through it for her, although I would have in an instant. I had thought of myself as the powerful family protector. Now I was defenseless against an unseen enemy that I knew only by two words: breast cancer. My wife was afraid she would soon face death, and I was worried too.

After a few minutes of sitting together at the breakfast bar and just being there for each other, we dried our eyes and gathered ourselves the best we could. She left for an appointment that she didn't want to be late for and I sat there, beginning to think of ways I could make this more bearable for her.

It was happening so fast.

Chapter 5

CELEBRATING WHILE STILL REELING

S till reeling from the diagnosis, we went to celebrate another birthday—for Phyllis' mother Doris—at The Cypress Inn Restaurant. It is situated on the Black Warrior River in Tuscaloosa not far from our home. We had a nice table with a window seat. We gazed admiringly down at the barges floating goods down river to the Gulf. We even saw the University of Alabama's rowing team practicing for a meet. It would have been perfect had it not been for the long shadow cast by the breast cancer diagnosis.

We were in uncharted territory. Together.

We gave Doris our presents and took a few pictures with the birthday girl. Throughout that dinner I made eye contact with Phyllis, sharing our secret and my support without saying a word. I needed her to know that she could count on me and she needed to know she wouldn't have to go through this alone. What exactly "this" was, neither of us knew. We were in uncharted territory. Together.

Chapter 6

MAGNETIC RESONANCE IMAGING (MRI)

We could only take one step at a time, and the following week Phyllis was scheduled for an MRI. I was dreading this for Phyllis because she is claustrophobic and an MRI requires that you lie on your back while they push your whole body into a tube-like machine that takes pictures of the internal workings of the body. This information would help the doctors to get the clearest picture of Phyllis' cancer. We knew that afterward there would be another stressful wait to learn the results of a test, which seemed to be the story of our life now.

She had her eyes closed, repeating the Lord's Prayer and 23 Psalm for twenty minutes until the test was complete.

At the DCH Hospital, Phyllis accepted the mild sedative the doctor offered and put on her thin hospital gown and cotton socks. I remember that she was cold and I was helpless to make her warm. I was leaving the room as they pushed her into the tube and the machine started thumping. She had her eyes closed, repeating the Lord's Prayer and 23 Psalm for twenty minutes until the test was complete. I made my way back to her as they slid her out of the tube. She looked over at me with her top lip quivering again—I nearly lost it then. The nurse said it was common to be emotional after an MRI and added, "You have a lot of time to think in there." Phyllis apologized for crying.

I had not been able to be with Phyllis during the biopsy, only being allowed in the recovery room, but during the MRI, they let me observe through the glass wall of the room where the clanking MRI machine was. She knew I was there, and if she began to panic I imagined going through that door and getting her out. I was beginning to find ways to help. We were in this together.

Chapter 7

CONSULTATION WITH ONCOLOGIST

The following week—just eleven days since we'd learned Phyllis had breast cancer—we made our way up to the second level of a five-level parking deck at the Lewis and Faye Manderson Cancer Center. I was taking Phyllis to get treatment recommendations from the oncologist. Of course, we knew Phyllis had breast cancer, but we were both still in denial. She would not even allow me to park in the reserved parking spaces for the patients of Manderson Cancer Center that were right at the entrance to the Center. She said, "That's for cancer patients." Seriously. So, we parked our car at the other end of the parking deck and made our way to the entrance of the Manderson Cancer Center.

As I went with Phyllis to visit Dr. Hinton we made what we thought of as our death march into the Manderson Cancer Center. For the first time, I was scared. I had no idea of what to expect except what I had heard from others or had read online, and none of that was anything to be happy about. I only knew one thing and that was that I had to be there with her. It was never a question with me of should I or should I not go. I was going because I knew I was the one Phyllis most wanted with her.

The waiting room was sizable, and as a real estate professional, I can't help but calculate square footage when I walk into a space. As I quietly did the math, I was puzzled. How could this much space be needed? I realized then what a big business cancer treatment has created. That huge room was filled with sad patients. Young, old, black, white, brown and yellow, proof that cancer isn't prejudiced. Illness is the ultimate equalizer.

I scanned the room for a couple of empty seats. One young lady in her early twenties sat there, wearing a colorful scarf around her head. She was flipping through a magazine with what looked like her mother accompanying her. In another seat, an older African-American gentleman waited with his aluminum walker. It had yellow tennis balls on the legs. He had a couple of male friends with him—maybe his sons. Then, there alone, sat a rail thin lady of about fifty years of age. The hopelessness in her eyes was gut-wrenching, and I had to look away.

My mind was screaming, "We don't belong in this place!" But it wasn't true. We did. My wife, Phyllis, had breast cancer, and there was nothing I could do about it. I needed to do something, anything, to get control of this situation. I consoled myself that at least I was with her today.

Phyllis took her number from the nice nurse at the front desk against the back wall and waited to be called. We anxiously sat there, keeping our thoughts to ourselves and not interested in any outdated magazines. It was not a long wait.

When her number was called, I went with her, not asking permission, taking the ask-for-forgiveness-later-if-needed approach. We walked through the large wooden double doors that opened into a twenty-feet wide corridor. To our left was the nurse's station that would start the prep work. They took her blood pressure, weight, name, insurance carrier, social security number, etc. After they finished the prep work, we were shown to an examination room with the usual exam table, two chairs, and supply cabinet. A strictly-business nurse soon joined us and peppered her with additional questions. We were going through the motions like zombies, but it wasn't as bad as the parking deck or waiting room. At least we were doing something.

The registered nurse finally finished with the hundred-question quiz and we were alone again. A gentle knock sounded at the door and in walked Dr. David Hinton. Phyllis had chosen Dr. Hinton as her oncologist, and it had been an easy choice. Besides being recognized as one of the top oncologists in our area, Dr. Hinton was our friend. His wife, Iris, worked with us as a Realtor at RE/MAX Premiere Group and we had met Dr. Hinton at numerous social events. His practice is an affiliate with M. D. Anderson Hospital in Houston, Texas, that is generally recognized as one of the top two hospitals in the country specializing in cancer care and research. With these credentials, we both felt Phyllis would be in good hands.

After a few pleasantries, Dr. Hinton got to the point. He was kind but direct. Phyllis needed to have a single mastectomy. The biopsy had confirmed the cancer was HER2 positive, which meant it was an aggressive type of cancer that just a few short years earlier had been extremely bad news, but a chemotherapy drug had been developed called Herceptin that had had tremendous results. Having the HER2 gene guaranteed the need for chemotherapy, regardless. Up until this point I guess I thought that maybe, just maybe, this would all go away and we would get back to our nice lives. Not this time. This was real life. One of the first reactions she

> *They were taking my wife's breast, and there was nothing I could do about it.*

had when Dr. Hinton said she would have to have chemotherapy was, "I will lose my hair, won't I?" They were taking my wife's breast, and there was nothing I could do about it.

Dr. Hinton candidly discussed with us her diagnosis and options. Would she have a single mastectomy or go ahead with a precautionary double mastectomy? Would she begin reconstructive surgery during or after the mastectomy? Would she even do reconstructive surgery at all? These choices were all ultimately Phyllis' decisions, and they were laid out to her in a few short minutes.

Phyllis sat there, as beautiful as ever (I married up, remember?), trying to be strong but I knew she was devastated. I thought my heart would break! I tried to be strong for her but I don't think I did a very good job that day.

> *She didn't break down in the exam room, but we agreed later that it was like an out-of-body experience for both of us.*

She didn't break down in the exam room, but we agreed later that it was like an out-of-body experience for both of us. Phyllis was attentive and hung on every detail the doctor had to offer, searching to hear something, anything, that would give her reason to be hopeful.

I was mostly focused on Phyllis and I remember thinking, "How could this be?" She seemed to be in excellent health! Her numbers were always perfect whenever she had a checkup. Blood pressure 120/75, low bad cholesterol, high good cholesterol, perfect weight to height ratio, and she ate salad and yogurt every day! Here I was overweight and, let's just say, lax on my good health habits, and here she was dealing with this crap when it should have been me. Yes, it should have been me instead of her. I really struggled with my lack of control of the situation and guilt that it wasn't me being diagnosed with cancer.

After hearing all of her options, Phyllis asked Dr. Hinton for his opinion. He recommended a single mastectomy, *if* she didn't test positive for the inherited gene that increases the risk of breast cancer. If she did, then she may want to consider a double mastectomy. The only way to find out was with a BRCA test.

The breast cancer (BRCA) gene test is a blood test to check for changes (mutations) in genes called BRCA1 and BRCA2. This test can help you know your chance of getting breast cancer and ovarian cancer. A BRCA gene test does not test for cancer itself. A woman's risk of breast and ovarian cancer is higher if she has BRCA1 or BRCA2 gene changes. Men with these gene changes also have a higher risk of breast cancer. And both men and women with these changes may be at higher risk for other cancers. You can inherit the gene changes from either your mother's or father's side of the family. This test is recommended for people with a strong family history of breast cancer or ovarian cancer or who already have one of these diseases. If none of these is true for you, you are not likely to have a BRCA gene change. Only about 2 or 3 out of 1,000 adult women have a BRCA gene change. That means 997 or 998 out of 1,000 women do not have this change. Phyllis asked Dr. Hinton if she needed to be tested for the gene, and he said it was her choice. She chose to forego this test but wondered aloud if she should encourage our daughter to have the BRCA test.

With all the information laid on her in the last half hour, Phyllis was inclined to go with Dr. Hinton's recommendation of a single mastectomy since the cancer appeared to be small and only in her left breast. She looked to me and asked me what I thought. I nodded. I was in full agreement with her decision. I was on autopilot now. The entire conversation with Dr. Hinton had left me somewhat numb, but I was thankful for the "cancer doctor" and his decisive comments based on his years of experience. I felt like he was part of our team or we were part of his. I couldn't decide which was which. I only knew I wasn't controlling the situation.

The conversation shifted to the actual surgery and what she could expect. Dr. Hinton was not a surgeon, so Phyllis needed to choose one. She chose the surgeon: Dr. Andy Harrell, who had performed the biopsy just a few days ago. Dr. Hinton explained that during surgery, Dr. Harrell would remove a few lymph nodes for test purposes. I sent up another prayer that this test would bring favorable results. Based on the results of the lymph nodes test, Dr. Hinton and his team would decide what level of treatment Phyllis needed. He was certain she would have chemotherapy and possibly radiation treatments if the lymph nodes were involved.

Phyllis decided to forego the reconstructive surgery at the time of the mastectomy. This would involve putting in what is called expanders that would push the skin away from the chest wall and prepare her for implants. Phyllis wanted to wait until after she was finished with her breast cancer treatments to make these decisions. It was just too much for her at that time. Again, I was in agreement because at the moment my only concern was killing the cancer in her body.

As the appointment was winding down, Dr. Hinton said he needed to check Phyllis' breast for any sudden changes over the last few days. I was not prepared for this. Men, your wife may be an exhibitionist, but I knew Phyllis wasn't. This was the first time I had been in the room while she had a breast exam with a male doctor. It was awkward for me because my inclination was to protect my wife from a man touching her breasts. I reminded myself that Dr. Hinton was a professional and that I could trust him. Early on, I had made up my own Rule #1: It's not about me. In the days and weeks to come this sense of modesty would pretty much go out the window. But at the time we both felt pretty uncomfortable, and this was about to become her new normal. We learned to laugh about how many male doctors and women saw her breasts through this ordeal. Or how many breasts she saw, since many former breast cancer survivors would later show Phyllis how well their reconstruction turned out.

This office visit was sure putting things in a sharp perspective. In one short hour, I had completely forgotten about all the real estate deals that previously consumed my thoughts. My attitude was changing. I was getting into fight mode. We now had a plan that would battle breast cancer, and I would find some way to help Phyllis fight this. I had no idea how, but I was determined to figure it out.

We left Manderson Cancer Center physically and emotionally drained, yet somehow better. At least we knew what we were dealing with. Our plan now was to be proactive, which was more in line with our personalities. Phyllis and I had never thought of ourselves as victims, and we would do everything in our power to beat this breast cancer. I would do my best. I just didn't know if my best would be enough.

The mastectomy was scheduled for August 5, 2014—all of eighteen days since we first learned Phyllis had breast cancer.

Chapter 8

SURGERY DAY

B y the time surgery day arrived, Phyllis had shared her bad news with immediate family and close friends. She was getting much-deserved sympathy but not enjoying it one bit. Phyllis had considered not telling anyone and keeping her diagnosis private, but that ship had sailed. She sadly said, "I'll be known now as the girl with breast cancer." She was private and was still struggling to acknowledge she had breast cancer.

I hated surgery day. Phyllis had prepared by buying beautiful silk pajamas to wear after the surgery. No tacky hospital gowns for her! She had been through all the tests, seen all the doctors, filled out all the insurance forms, and answered every question imaginable. It was time for them to take my wife's breast.

Then, hopped up on adrenaline, I would now have to sit and wait, feeling helpless to protect my wife from pain and suffering.

There had been so much stress around getting to that moment. We couldn't even see beyond it. Then, hopped up on adrenaline, I would now have to sit and wait, feeling helpless to protect my wife from pain and suffering. Would they come out and tell me that the cancer had spread to other parts of her body? Only time would tell. I prayed so much that morning.

We stayed in pre-op for a good amount of time while the nurses did their jobs. The main task at hand was to mark the *correct* breast and not the *right* breast. *Correct* being the important word here because it was her left breast that was cancerous. We had heard of surgeons operating on the wrong body part before, so "left" became the word of the day.

> *I felt I had failed her somehow by not being able to stop all this hurt.*

I was at peace with Phyllis having her breast removed but I found it hard to look her in the eyes. I felt I had failed her somehow by not being able to stop all this hurt. Phyllis seemed at peace too with what was about to transpire and was ready to get on with it. Ready to get on the road to recovery, but this gruesome task had to be done first.

Dr. Harrell came in to make sure the correct breast was marked. She was marked up like a conference room whiteboard with all the lines, circles, and arrows. Then the anesthesiologist came in and introduced himself and let her know what he would be responsible for. I was watching everyone like a hawk, kidding myself that I would know if they did anything incorrect when our old friend Kathy Givhan came in and informed us she would be the nurse anesthetist. We were both happy about that because we knew her to be thorough, precise, and intelligent. I relaxed a tiny bit, trusting she would keep everyone on task in the operating room.

The anesthesiologist gave Phyllis what he called "happy juice" to relax her, and just like that she was on her way. We said our goodbyes with a kiss, and they rolled her off to the operating room. She was already asleep, and I watched her until she was out of sight. Then I was alone.

Phyllis and I were never one of those couples who need to be together constantly. We have separate offices at work; occasionally we take separate vacations simply to have our alone time, and it works well for our relationship. I must say, though, I had separation anxiety on surgery day.

The Tuscaloosa DCH Hospital waiting room has 53 chairs (I counted), one television, and two monitors. I was restless and changed seats several times that day. I remember thinking about how many thousand rumps that had sat on these seats, waiting to hear news of a loved one, hoping it would be good. I couldn't get interested in the daytime talk show on the television or any news on social media. I did respond to a few texts from friends asking about Phyllis and me. I was not alone in my wait. Phyllis' fan club included my son Russell, daughter Caroline, Phyllis' mother Doris, sister-in-law Michelle, and Phyllis' sister Becky. DCH did have a good system of informing family and friends with monitors throughout the waiting room with updates on the surgery's progress using the patient's number onscreen for privacy. That let me know when the surgery had begun, when it was over, and when she was in the recovery room. I liked that. It kept us in the loop. Otherwise I think I'd have gone nuts.

Soon I heard my name being called to meet with Dr. Harrell. What was I about to hear? I knew many prayers had gone up for my wife that day, and I had faith all would be well. I met Dr. Harrell in a small private cubicle that had a couple of chairs. One of the many forms Phyllis had signed before surgery gave her permission for Dr. Harrell to share any and all of her medical information with me. He informed me that everything went "great" and they only had to take out two lymph nodes for testing purposes and that none others looked involved. It looked like the cancer had not spread, but we would not know for sure until the tests results came back. So, we would have another test result to wait on.

He then explained the drains. Somehow before this moment I had totally missed the conversation regarding the drains. A mastectomy is such a radical surgery with the severing of so many blood vessels that drains were needed to keep the fluids from building up and pooling beneath the incision. These drains had to be emptied and the contents measured for several days after the mastectomy. I was a little horrified to hear about this. It reminded me of what an invasion to Phyllis' body the surgery was. It was an amputation. I was energized, though, at the news that there was a task for me at last! I finally had a job—something I could do to help.

We stayed overnight in a private hospital room at Tuscaloosa DCH. Phyllis received excellent one-on-one care from the nurses. It wasn't an Intensive Care Unit, but I felt like Phyllis was a celebrity with the care she received that night. True to her nature, Phyllis, with the help of the pain meds, was trying to get up, move around, and put on some makeup. I was so relieved that she wasn't in pain. I stayed with her that night resting in a somewhat comfortable recliner, not sleeping much with the attentive nursing staff frequently monitoring her vitals.

By the next morning the zero-pain anesthesia had almost worn off, and Phyllis was now depending on oral pain medications, which were doing a fair job. We waited on Dr. Harrell to make his rounds, and he arrived around 8:00 a.m. The doctor unwrapped the tightly-wound bandage that was compressing her chest. This was the first time I had seen the results of the surgery. I had prepared myself by looking online at mastectomy pictures, but this was the first time I had seen my wife's wounded chest. The incision was horizontal. Tubes drained the excess blood and fluids into a plastic bag that measured the exact amount. I was having mixed emotions: happy with the successful surgery but broken-hearted that Phyllis refused to look down at her chest. She looked anywhere else as the doctor checked her incision and drains. She just wasn't ready to see the damage yet. She would choose when her first look would be. A while later, she went into the bathroom alone, locked the door, and checked her new self out. I let her have her privacy and after a few minutes she emerged without commenting. I didn't push her for words.

Dr. Harrell tightly wrapped her again and gave us his instructions on how to care for the wound and said we could go home. In my opinion, when you have a part of your body cut off, you should stay under the care of the experts longer than overnight. However, due to the fact that the insurance companies think they know more about health care than doctors and because they have to keep their bottom line in check, you can't stay longer than the mighty insurance companies' decree.

We signed a few discharge papers, and I gathered our personal items from the room as the nurse situated Phyllis in the wheelchair. The insurance companies that insist you should leave one day after a major surgery refuse to let you walk out of the hospital on your own. Crazy. I held the door as the nurse wheeled her through the crowded waiting room. Phyllis looked like a celebrity that morning, and I guess the crowd thought I was her bodyguard. They had no idea how true that was.

We were happy to be on our way home, and I began my new adventure at being Phyllis' nurse. I had her pillows propped up on the bed like she liked them, and as soon as we arrived she laid down. By now the anesthesia from the surgery had totally worn off and she was in pain and nauseated,

> *She was watching my reaction the entire time to see if she could read any disappointment in my eyes.*

which was expected. What wasn't expected was the huge black and blue bubble forming underneath the incision.

At midday, I was on my maiden voyage of nursing Phyllis back to good health. We were in our bathroom as I measured and recorded the amount of fluid that had drained into the bags under her chest compression wrap. I got a good look at her scar for the first time when I helped empty the drains that were needed to relieve any fluid buildup from the surgery. She was watching my reaction the entire time to see if she could read any disappointment in my eyes. I realized at that moment she would always be beautiful to me, and I hoped it showed. I think it did. We looked at the results of the mastectomy together. She asked how I thought it looked. I was honest and told her it was different but added I thought she was still a keeper. It was harder for Phyllis to allow me to see her empty chest than it was for her to look herself.

The bags were full, and a sizable dark blue pocket had formed below the incision. We wondered if this was normal. I decided it wasn't or the doctor would have mentioned the possibility of this happening. Not taking any chances, I took the initiative and called Dr. Harrell's office. He informed me that the pooling was not normal and it was most likely a hematoma. He wanted me to bring her to the Emergency Room at DCH Hospital. So, after a few short hours at home the day after surgery, Phyllis was on her way back to the hospital.

Chapter 9

EMERGENCY ROOM VISIT

Caroline took her mother to the Emergency Room while I took care of getting her prescriptions filled and catching up on a few other issues that required my attention. My family knows how to work as a team. Caroline called to let me know when Dr. Harrell had joined them at the ER and examined Phyllis. He determined that he needed to go back in and repair the leaking blood vessels that were causing the hematoma. Phyllis was to have two surgeries in two days!

No one was happy. Dr. Harrell wasn't happy about having to put his patient through another surgery, but there was no other alternative. I was fighting hard to keep my temper in check and trying to

I was fighting hard to keep my temper in check and trying to remember Rule #1: It's not about me.

remember Rule #1: It's not about me. Phyllis was furious! She was angry for having to go through another surgery and wasn't real concerned who knew it.

Back to Surgery

Breast Surgery, Part Two was scheduled for late that afternoon. Phyllis was sent directly to pre-op to begin the process of getting prepped for another surgery. Prepping for the second surgery wasn't as involved as the first one. No drawing or marking up of the area. Everyone knew exactly the area that needed attention. Prepping was basically keeping Phyllis calm. She had been agitated because she doesn't like surprises and had been in pain the entire day, which made for a long afternoon for Caroline! At some point, Caroline crawled into Phyllis' bed and was praying with her when Caroline's stomach growled. That's when Phyllis' frustrations were replaced with worry that her "baby" was hungry! At least it got her mind off the other problem and gave her something else to be mad about. When I arrived, I found myself in the role reversal of tempering my wife's temper for once. She calmed down, knowing I would take care of Caroline and the situation.

After going through the limited prepping process again, we had to wait a while for Dr. Harrell. It was quiet as the nurses were out of things to say. I snapped out of my daze to notice how the medical professionals in the room looked like a biker gang with do-rags on their heads. I kept these thoughts to myself, not wanting to say anything negative to the people that were taking care of my wife. Finally, the leader of the gang, Dr. Harrell and his assistant arrived with their do-rags and warm lab coats on. Phyllis was still concerned and agitated that her baby Caroline was hungry and cold.

Dr. Harrell started explaining all things related to the second surgery. Phyllis was giving him a look that held no compassion. I had been on the receiving end of the same look from her and her father. She asked Dr. Harrell if she would be getting a discount this time, and she was not kidding. We had excellent health insurance, but she couldn't help complaining about health care costs. I think she rightly thought that spending that much money should at least be hassle-free, if not pleasant. The meds to get her started for Breast Surgery, Part Two were administered and thankfully she mellowed slightly, but as the drugs took effect, she calmly cursed the doctor while telling a random story about chickens. Go figure.

The second surgery was a success. Oddly enough, I was more relaxed the second go-round than during the previous day's surgery. I told Phyllis later that she probably received the best care of her life the evening of Breast Surgery, Part Two. Everyone was hyper-focused trying to avoid any mistakes. We stayed another night at the hospital—both of us sleeping fitfully. I was ready for my own bed but certainly not complaining. Then the next morning she was discharged once again. I think we both thought we were pros by this time.

Discharged . . . Again

Phyllis was sent home with an extremely tight compression wrap around her chest. The drains dangled underneath the wrap and were very cumbersome. She felt them every time she rolled over or moved in bed. Finally, with enough pain meds, she was able to rest somewhat comfortably. I must have walked into our bedroom a thousand times to check on her those first few days. Many times, I stood quietly in the doorway, just watching her chest rise and fall, making sure she was still breathing. My wife was home, and all was well.

Back to Work

A few days later and predictably, my hard-working wife was eager to get back to work. She was still on pain meds and wasn't supposed to drive, but I learned long ago that when it came to work, Phyllis would not be stopped. Besides, working is good medicine. Those who work and stay productive don't have time for self-pity. Several friends had volunteered to help her out. She said she had always wanted a chauffeur, so she took them up on their offers.

Phyllis' assistant and future daughter-in-law, Amanda, chauffeured her to Kyle Stationary to get the thank-you cards she had ordered to send to everyone that had called or that had sent get well soon cards. With drains dangling, Phyllis moaned at every bump in the road, but she was adamant about those thank-you cards. She said it would give her something to do while recuperating.

Chapter 10

WHAT DID KEN SAY?

Amidst the frenzy of the diagnosis and surgeries, Phyllis and I were doing well to put one foot in front of the other. There wasn't a lot of time for reflection or philosophizing. Even so, it seemed like everyone who heard about Phyllis' ordeal wanted to talk about our thoughts and feelings. Phyllis told me that the first question out of women's mouths when they heard her news was, "What did Ken say?" This seemed to be a little shortsighted and perhaps insensitive to me at first, but I quickly realized that this question came from a place of true empathy. Our friends wanted to be assured that Phyllis could depend on me now more than ever. After all, I was thinking the same thing. I wanted Phyllis to know she could depend on me, no matter what. That's when I came up with my Rule #1 for life after a breast cancer diagnosis: "It's not about me!" From that moment forward, it was all about her. It was about getting her through this ordeal with the least amount of worries and regrets. This was no easy task. Change is hard.

Men and women alike will go to great lengths to avoid change. We get in our comfort zones and don't want to leave them. That's why they're called comfort zones, but breast cancer will force you out of them.

I've always considered myself pretty helpful around the house. Over the years we had figured out who did what best and without ever saying, "That's your job!" We simply did the chore each did the best. I was in charge of the yard chores, cutting the lawn, trimming hedges, fertilizing, etc. Phyllis loved to putter around outside too. She usually did our laundry, but I knew how to separate clothes and turn on the washing machine and if I needed something washed, I did it myself. We both cooked dinner, and usually the one who made it home first was in charge that night. But after her surgeries, I took charge of it all or, for a while, at least. She wasn't helpless, but I tried to do the heavy lifting as much as possible. It didn't take long for me to realize she had been doing a lot more than me around the house!

I made it my mindset to just do it if it needed doing. It was all about her getting through this with the least amount of stress.

Post-op

When Phyllis was discharged, we learned that it would take a few weeks for her wounds to heal. She would need my help emptying the drains for ten days after the surgery. Did that slow her down? No way. On the advice from friends who had recently gone through a mastectomy, she'd bought a few loose-fitting blouses that would hide the drains. She went to the office, showed houses, and persevered without complaint. After a few days of being carted around by friends, Phyllis decided her dream of having a chauffeur was overrated and began driving again. Even today she will tell you that staying busy was her saving grace. She forced herself to get up, get dressed, put on some lipstick and a smile and move forward instead of staying home feeling sorry for herself. She embraced the opportunity to stay positive and show joy. As I quietly observed, my respect for her grew.

On August 14, Dr. Harrell removed the drains. I realize that may seem a little thing to some, but it was an important landmark for her. I felt a small victory at having helped her to that point. I had been engaged in the first process of surgery and assisting with the drains, so I was proud to say I had helped.

As I quietly observed, my respect for her grew.

My biggest challenge was to get her to take it easy. She was beginning to feel better and was getting accustomed to the new Phyllis, and it showed. Not happy with the change but accepting it. Just three days after the drains came out, she flew with her Tuscaloosa Association of Realtors Executive, Nikki Simmons, to Chicago for a National Association of Realtors convention wearing her compression sleeve during the flight because of the risk of lymphedema, a condition that sometimes causes swelling in the arms after lymph nodes removal. Even though this was not a problem for Phyllis, to this day, whenever I see a woman with one arm swollen from lymphedema, I empathize with what she's been through or is going through. I stayed home, and we both got a much-needed break from our post-op routine.

Chapter 11

THE SCANS

Positron Emission Tomography (PET) Scan

When she got home from her Chicago trip, Phyllis went alone (she considered herself a big girl now) to Tuscaloosa DCH. There she was injected with radioactive glucose for her PET Scan. Many cancer cells will quickly synthesize with the radioactive glucose, and this allows the physician, through the scan, to locate the site of the cancer and determine its size. It also will differentiate benign from malignant growths and discover if the cancer is spreading. This assists the physician in selecting the best or least invasive treatments and monitors the success of the chosen therapy. Once the injection was fully engaged, she was slid into another machine, not like the closed-in MRI machine but more open, where her full body was scanned. Dr. Hinton now had a 3-D picture that gave him a baseline to gauge her future progress.

Her next appointment was two days later, after the PET Scan, with Dr. Hinton at the Manderson Cancer Center. By now we knew the drill of driving up the parking deck, parking at the far end, taking a number, and waiting our turn in a room filled mostly with patients in despair. This time when her number was called, we went directly back to an examination room and waited for Dr. Hinton. She sat on the exam table, and I took my place in the corner chair.

Dr. Hinton came in and gave us the good news. The results of the PET Scan were great! No other cancer was found in her body! This was a big deal, and I breathed a huge sigh of relief. Since she had tested HER2 positive, Dr. Hinton said that chemotherapy treatment was a must.

It was hard for me to follow the rationale of needing further treatments if no cancer was in her body . . .

HER2/neu (shortened to HER2) is a growth-promoting protein on the outside of all breast cells. Breast cancer cells with the higher than normal levels of HER2 are called HER2-positive. These cancers tend to grow and spread faster than other breast cancers. That's why all women newly diagnosed with invasive breast cancers are tested for HER2.

Wait, didn't I just hear him say that the cancer was gone? It was hard for me to follow the rationale of needing further treatments if no cancer was in her body, but Dr. Hinton said it would be malpractice on his part if he didn't insist she have chemotherapy. I said early on that I would have to depend on the experts and this was one of the times. Phyllis decided she would begin chemotherapy on the doctor's advice, and I was certainly on board with her decision.

Multigated Acquisition Scan (MUGA) Scan

A few days later on August 25th, she had to have another test called a MUGA scan to determine if Phyllis' heart was strong enough for treatment. MUGA Scan is a noninvasive diagnostic test used to evaluate the pumping function of the ventricles (lower chambers of the heart). It was another important baseline test that would measure the effects of the chemotherapy on her heart. During the test, a small amount of radioactive tracer is injected into a vein. A special camera, called a gamma camera, detects the radiation released by the tracer to produce computer-generated movie images of the beating heart.[1]

The MUGA Scan was performed at Tuscaloosa DCH Imaging, and Phyllis informed me this was a fairly easy procedure much like a regular doctor visit so I found something to do at my office. She came to the office when it was over and said it was "easy peasy."

---

1   https://myclevelandclinic.org

Chapter 12

GATLINBURG RETREAT

W hen Phyllis was recovering from her mastectomy surgery, I'd wake in the middle of the night, and my first thought would be, "My wife has breast cancer." When I'd wake in the morning, my mind immediately registered, breast cancer. It was difficult to compartmentalize and stay focused on the tasks of my daily life with this looming large in my mind. I had to work hard not to bore other people with my breast cancer talk, and I also figured it unlikely that anyone would be interested in how I'd mastered drainage care!

Even though cancer can feel like a lonely journey, I was pleasantly surprised at the support group that began to grow for Phyllis and me. Our support group included a dear friend by the name of Jimmy Kuykendall or as we called him, BoBo. Jimmy and his wife Janice lived nearby in Tuscaloosa, and we had been friends for forty years. Jimmy was also fighting cancer at the time and was taking many trips to M. D. Anderson in Houston, Texas. The side effects of the aggressive treatments he was taking were harsh but you would never know it because he and Janice stayed on the go, traveling all over the United States.

Phyllis told Janice about her diagnosis early on, and Janice immediately started planning a time we would visit them at their Smoky Mountain retreat in Gatlinburg, Tennessee. We decided the ideal time would be after Phyllis' mastectomy and before her chemo treatments. I was fine with whatever dates they decided on because I was living by my Rule #1 and I was ready to head north for cooler weather anyway.

Phyllis and I took the interstate highways most of the way, and I had plenty of time to think while driving since Phyllis was staring down at her telephone and iPad the entire trip. Driving is where I usually solved the world's problems, but I was a little apprehensive about the visit. I didn't want to make Jimmy uncomfortable by asking about his cancer fight but on the flipside, I didn't want him to think I wasn't concerned. I relaxed and told myself he was just my old friend, and I'd talk about what he wanted to talk about. I applied Rule #1 to him too.

When we turned onto Highway 441 in Knoxville, Tennessee, we could feel we were getting close to the Great Smoky Mountains. We were leaving the gentle landscape the Tennessee Highway Department had created when building their interstate and started seeing in the distance the smoky mountains that defined the area. We stayed on Highway 441 through Pigeon Forge, home of Dollywood owned by the tough businesswoman Dolly Parton. We turned onto Highway 321, which led us to Gatlinburg the self-proclaimed gateway to the Great Smoky Mountains. We marveled at how Gatlinburg had changed since we last visited twenty years ago and how it had become very commercialized and touristy.

With the help of GPS, I found the street that lead to Janice and Jimmy's cabin. We arrived to find a nice, modern home built on stilts in a mountain subdivision with the Little Pigeon River flowing in their backyard. They came out and greeted us before we got out of the car, and paying no attention to the time lapse since we last saw them, our conversations took up where we had left them off months ago. It's like that with old friends. Going up the steps with our overnight bags, Phyllis and I stopped to admire Jimmy's 1957 Bel Air Chevrolet red convertible parked underneath the house in the carport that was created by the stilts. You could see your reflection in the deep-mirrored finish. Jimmy told us he'd restored the car himself and had hauled it to Gatlinburg on his car trailer to enter it in the Pigeon Forge Car Show that weekend. Thousands of fans and participants would soon line both sides of the parkway to admire the hot rods ripping up and down the road or just to take a stroll on the sidewalk viewing the classic cars in their favorite parking spaces facing the parkway. Many simply set up their tents and coolers to enjoy the show going by, remembering the first time they had seen this or that particular model. I regretted that our schedule had us leaving before the show began, but we saw many of the classic cars anyway.

After we settled in our bedroom, we met in the kitchen/den combination. We reminisced and laughed about old times. Forty years ago, Jimmy had taught Phyllis and me how to water-ski on Lake Tuscaloosa, behind his Glastron walk-through windshield boat that had a 115-horse power Johnson motor. A walk-through has a windshield with a section that hinges in the middle that allows you to walk through to the front seats of the boat. It took *all* 115 horses to pull me up on that Dick Pope slalom ski. I can still see Jimmy sitting on his knees, making it easier for him to watch us in case we fell or wiped out. Those were good times with very few real-life concerns. We would launch our boats at Buster Tierce's Marina and float just around the bend to the waterfront lots we rented from Mr. Buster Tierce. Sometimes we went to the lake on Friday after work, then again on Saturday morning and stayed until dark and hit the water again on Sunday afternoon. Occasionally on Sunday afternoon we would leave the water early enough to get all our gang together at the Catfish Cabin on Jug Factory Road in Tuscaloosa. Larry, Teresa, Claude, Teresa (Diego), Jackie, Jennifer, Greg, and Cindy were happy to join us. They served sweet tea by the quart glass and all the slaw, hush puppies, and whole fried catfish you could eat. We always got our money's worth there.

Phyllis and Janice laughed about Jimmy's big-boy toys and how I tended to emulate his spending habits. Jimmy had a boat; I bought a boat Jimmy found for me. Jimmy had a van; I bought a van Jimmy found for me. Jimmy had a Corvette; I bought a Corvette Jimmy found for me. Ah, my 1979, L82 little red Corvette! I loved that car, and I kept it spotless! I had to sell it when Phyllis was pregnant with our first child because I couldn't figure out a way to get the car seat to cooperate. I learned to be careful mentioning anything on my wish list to Jimmy because if I did, he'd go out and find it and then negotiate the best price for me. He loved helping me spend my money! We reminisced about all these things and embellished greatly on the trip. I was reminded why they always say laughter is good medicine. I don't know why I had been anxious on the drive up.

The conversation finally turned serious when Phyllis and Jimmy started talking about their cancer issues. They asked each other what was next, and when Phyllis told Jimmy she would be starting chemotherapy in a few days, he grimaced. He knew what she was about to go through and knew better than most that it would not be pleasant, so he shared a little of his prognosis with her. His cancer had started in his thyroid, and he then developed a tumor on his spine. But he was positive that the trips to Houston were keeping the cancer in check.

The next morning, we woke up to Janice cooking her typical breakfast for Jimmy. She had hot biscuits for us to spoon Jimmy's favorite mixture of Golden Eagle Table Syrup and peanut butter on. We used to tease Janice that she had spoiled Jimmy rotten and that was *before* he got cancer! Now it was almost ridiculous, but I could understand it completely because I was living that life too now.

After breakfast, Phyllis wanted to fish in the Little Pigeon River so we both wet a hook. Wetting a hook was all we accomplished because the fish were not biting. But standing on the grassy bank while watching the current take whatever bothered to float downstream was very peaceful.

As sick as Jimmy was, he and Janice made sure they were good hosts to their houseguests, and after fishing a while, we piled in Jimmy's truck to visit Gatlinburg for lunch and to walk through the shops. That money-grabbing excursion being completed and a good lunch in our bellies, we decided to take a quick road trip through Cades Cove, the old self-sustaining farm nestled in a tranquil valley just outside of Gatlinburg. We saw dozens of classic car owners out enjoying the day like us. Phyllis and I both mused that we would have loved to be in Jimmy's 57 Chevy, but it was show-ready spotless and he didn't want to get it dirty and have to detail it again. He had several trophies that proved he knew what it took to win a Classic Car Show trophy.

The trip through Cades Cove took longer than expected with the heavy traffic from the car show enthusiasts, and we got stuck in the slow parade of cars winding their way through the nature lover's cove. We were in good company, and we were looking for black bears so the slow traffic wasn't so bad.

We stayed another night, then rose early so we could get on the road. We didn't want to overstay our welcome, and they had a car show to attend.

As we were making our way back to Tuscaloosa, Phyllis shared that Janice whispered to her that Jimmy had had a rough night. The medicine he was trying was upsetting to his digestive system, and he had stayed in the bathroom all night. He never let on that he had any problems the morning we left, but that was Bobo—not seeking any sympathy or seeing the need to make us feel uncomfortable.

Phyllis said, "Jimmy and Janice are determined to keep living, in spite of it all."

Visiting with them that short weekend in Gatlinburg inspired Phyllis to face her breast cancer with a renewed determination, and it inspired me because Jimmy was a good friend and I was proud of him for being brave in the face of such a frightening disease. Janice was such a willing caregiver and refused to let her husband fight alone, so I reaffirmed my resolve to be there for my wife, too, and try, in my limited capacity, to ease some of the pain and stress that was ahead.

I reaffirmed my resolve to be there for my wife, too, and try, in my limited capacity, to ease some of the pain and stress that was ahead.

Our trip home from Gatlinburg was so nice. We turned off our electronic devices for a while and allowed ourselves to have an original thought not dictated by what was on social media. We took the opportunity to clear our minds for the next step in this journey.

Jimmy Kuykendall lost his battle with cancer on April 19, 2017, at the age of sixty-six. He and Janice endured his disease and subsequent death in the most dignified manner I have ever witnessed. The way he chose to live his last few years on this earth was rewarded with friends speaking at his funeral service and sharing stories of their time together that sounded much like my experiences with Jimmy. Cancer didn't beat Jimmy. He went out on his terms. The long line of classic cars in the funeral procession paid tribute to the passion he loved.

I know there has to be a section in Heaven where they have car shows, and I believe Jimmy's there now.

Chapter 13
MEDIPORT

The Tuesday following our Gatlinburg trip, Phyllis was scheduled for outpatient surgery to install a mediport, which is a small medical appliance placed beneath the skin. I was beginning to feel that everyone in the medical profession thought of my wife as an automobile. Send her through the drive-thru and install this or take off that. I didn't like that, but the experts said the mediport was better than trying to find a vein each time she required an injection, namely during chemotherapy. A mediport is much like a catheter that connects the port to a vein. Just under the skin, the port has a septum through which drugs can be injected and blood samples can be drawn many times, usually with less discomfort for the patient than a more typical "needle prick". Mediports are used mostly to treat hematology and oncology patients. The port is usually inserted in the upper chest, just below the clavicle or collarbone, leaving the patient's hands unencumbered during treatments.

The procedure went well, as expected. I felt proud of Phyllis for being such a trooper. She was proving to be an excellent patient. The next day, I worked at the office while Phyllis had a follow-up appointment with Dr. Hinton regarding the installed mediport.

> *I was beginning to feel that everyone in the medical profession thought of my wife as an automobile.*

He confirmed the mediport was good to go, and Phyllis agreed to schedule her chemotherapy treatments on Thursdays, planning it so she would have a chance to recuperate through the weekend so she could be back at work on Monday. This plan meant she would begin the journey we had been dreading *the very next day*. We were both eager to get the chemo behind us but anxious about the side effects.

Chapter 14

CHEMOTHERAPY

The time had come to start the chemotherapy treatments. After many hours of researching the process of the treatments, the names of the chemotherapy drugs Dr. Hinton would be using to treat Phyllis, and what their side effects would be, I had come away pretty much horrified. Chemotherapy can cure cancer, control cancer, or shrink tumors causing a person pain or pressure. The goal in Phyllis' case was to kill any undetected cancer cells since the PET Scan had shown no cancer in her body after the mastectomy. But the truth is that chemotherapy was going to kill many cells in my wife's body. The goal is to kill only the bad cells but some good cells would die too. I didn't want *any* part of Phyllis to die! But this was the choice Phyllis had made based on the expertise of Dr. Hinton, and we would stick to the plan. Rule #1 for me.

There is a long list of Chemotherapy drugs available that are case-specific to the individual's type of cancer and their health condition. The drugs Phyllis would be treated with were Paclitaxel (Taxol), Carboplatin,

> *The goal is to kill only the bad cells but some good cells would die too. I didn't want **any** part of Phyllis to die!*

and Herceptin. The side effects of these drugs were a laundry list of horror. Taxol: bruising, bleeding, reduced number of red blood cells, nausea, diarrhea, sore mouth, numbness in hands or feet, tiredness, hair loss, muscle and joint pain, dry skin and brittle nails. Carboplatin: all the above plus reduction in white blood cells that increases your risk of infection, constipation, loss of appetite, and sore mouth. Herceptin: flu-like symptoms, fever, chills, and possible heart damage. What a list!

In many cases, radiation is used as a treatment in conjunction with the chemotherapy. Dr. Hinton had determined that Phyllis did not need radiation in addition to chemo, and that was welcome news since we'd learned radiation can burn the skin while killing the cancer cells.

In my pre-breast cancer life, I had few real worries. I enjoyed my family, going to work, helping the agents at my company, going on the occasional vacation, reading, and cooking. But after everything we had been through, I suddenly realized we had created new habits centering around what was next on the treating-breast-cancer list, and we had gotten accustomed to our routine. Crazy as it may sound, we had gotten comfortable again. It had been thirty days since her mastectomy, and Phyllis was feeling much better physically. The horizontal incision on her chest had healed nicely. We marveled at the healing power of the body along with prayer, which gave us hope for the days and weeks to come. But the day to start chemo had come, and that would start the process of her hair falling out. It was a big deal and was probably Phyllis' number two concern ranking behind survival, of course.

I had been committed from day one of the breast cancer diagnosis to help Phyllis in any way I possibly could, but after our Gatlinburg retreat, I'd recommitted that we would do this breast cancer thing together—doctor visits, treatments, and follow-ups. It was the least I could do, and as her husband, I'd try to keep my promise to support her in sickness and in health. Such a little thing, being there, but I could tell it meant the world to her.

So, I drove Phyllis to her early appointment at the Lewis and Faye Manderson Cancer Center. Dr. Hinton had warned us it would be an all-day affair, so we came prepared with our reading material (real estate contracts and laptops). It was a quiet ride again, much like the initial visit with Dr. Hinton, as we circled up to the second level of the parking deck, which was the entrance to the Manderson Cancer Center. The deck was about 75 percent full, and when we were close to the entrance of MCC, I spotted the vacant parking spaces reserved for Manderson Cancer Center patients. But we drove on past them and again she said, "Those are for the cancer patients." That was still funny to me, but that's my wife!

Side-by-side we walked into the waiting room. We walked past a display case advertising cheerful pink scarfs, prosthetic bras, prosthetic bra inserts, and pink hats that were available from the women's breast cancer volunteer group. I said, "I believe I could find a better place for that display." She agreed. The spacious waiting room was filled with a variety of patients. Some who waited looked frail, some were alone, a few had head coverings, some were obese, and some were very thin. No one was smiling. Manderson Cancer Center tried to make it as pleasant as possible with their floor-to-ceiling windows, professional décor, and the friendliest nurse out front, but most of the people waiting were there for chemotherapy treatments and this was serious business.

Phyllis gave the nurse her name, took a number again, and sat down to wait. "Number thirty-seven?" they called. I quietly appreciated how they respected her privacy by not calling out her name. At the same time, it was strange that her intensely personal fight had been reduced to a numeric digit. It was surreal.

From the doctors to the support staff, all the folks at Manderson Cancer Center had given us every reason to relax in their care, but that day I felt jumpy and defensive like we were entering enemy territory. This place signified cancer and death to me. I had to remind myself of Rule #1 more than once. I prayed for peace and the right words to support and encourage my wife.

We then walked through big double doors for the first of eighteen weekly scheduled treatments. Phyllis stopped by the nurse's station on the left to have her vitals taken, and we were soon on our way to the treatment room at the end of the hall. There was a good deal of activity in the area and I thought, a lot of folks would be out of a job if it wasn't for cancer!

We entered the treatment room that I can only describe as an auditorium. Several rows of recliners faced personal televisions. *So far, so good,* I thought. *Now, if only these things have ESPN!* Phyllis was shown to her treatment station, which was on the second row from the back and close to a large window overlooking the terrace that was filled with large planters of shrubs and greenery. She had a neighbor on one side taking treatments, but I still felt as though she had her own space. Everything the patient and nurse needed was in this space except what I called the nuclear medicine. Even with all the amenities and personal preparations Manderson Cancer Center made, both Phyllis and I felt as if we didn't belong there. Imagining at any moment someone should be rushing in and exclaiming, "Wait! There's been a mistake. This room is just for sick people. Phyllis Olive isn't supposed to be here!"

Nurse Tammy sat down with her and began explaining the process and what she could expect the first day. After all the poking, prodding, and blood work, it was time to begin the actual chemotherapy treatment, administered through the mediport. At 10:00 a.m. on September 4—

forty-eight days from the day she first heard the diagnosis from Dr. Harrell—the Taxol, Carboplatin, and Herceptin entered her body. Phyllis' treatment schedule was three drugs the first day followed by a one-drug treatment the following Thursday and another one-drug treatment the Thursday after that. Then the cycle would start over with the three-drug treatment.

The registered nurses that were required to administer the chemo drugs, as prescribed by Dr. Hinton, both came in wearing thick, heavy masks and gloves. They held bags of fluid with all sorts of warnings on them. They then each had to sign off on the procedure immediately because the drugs they managed were deadly. Taxol, Carboplatin, and Herceptin, with all their side effects, were on the way into my wife's body to kill a part of her and I was worried about how her body would react to them.

Throughout the morning, they brought Phyllis all the juice and crackers she wanted but at lunch I went to Schlotzsky's and brought back an original for us to split, and it was delicious to us both.

I'll never forget how late that afternoon she started shivering like she was outside without a coat in the dead of winter. Not violently, but she could not control it. I was concerned to say the least, but it was nothing the nurses had not seen before. They called Dr. Hinton, he prescribed a Benadryl, and soon she was back to normal. I wondered how many women suffered the shaking during chemo before someone discovered that the common drug Benadryl would stop it.

Trying to pass the time that first day proved difficult for me. I was not accustomed to the surroundings, and I tend to be restless until I familiarize myself to a new place. I read, looked at my cell phone, and observed the busy activity of the treatment room and its patients. Phyllis did the same while thinking about the side effects of hair loss, nausea, vomiting, loss of appetite, and fatigue from the drugs now entering her body.

All the cancer-fighting drugs had made their way into her body by around 6:00 p.m., but it was one treatment down and seventeen treatments to go. The stress of experiencing chemotherapy for the first time as patient and caregiver had been eye-opening for both of us. It had been a very long day, and we were both exhausted. I prayed the side effects would be minimal. I considered myself fortunate to be with my wife that first day, but I felt as if I had just been the sole eyewitness to a heinous crime.

Neulasta

The next morning, feeling pretty good, Phyllis went back to MCC to get her Neulasta shot, or as her friend Kim Wolbach (also a breast cancer survivor) called it, "The New Nasty." One side effect of Neulasta is that it can make your bones ache horribly and is given to the patient twenty-four hours after receiving the chemo treatment. Neulasta made Kim's bones ache but did not affect Phyllis as much. Neulasta itself isn't a chemotherapy drug but is a medicine that is used to stimulate the growth of healthy white blood cells in the bone marrow, counteracting one of the side effects of Carboplatin, which is that it destroys white blood cells. Dr. Hinton had prescribed the Neulasta to help protect Phyllis' body against the infection risks while on the chemotherapy cycle. By this point, in an attempt to keep up, I started to write down all the names of the drugs. Anyone who can remember all the names of all the drugs and what they do without a list is likely a Mensa candidate or certainly deserves a gold star!

Side Effects

That afternoon after the Neulasta shot, everything took a turn for the worse. The previous day's chemotherapy drugs had started their "seek-and-destroy" mission. Phyllis became flushed, weak, and nauseated. I knew from experience that when Phyllis is nauseated, she wants to be left alone. She will not talk to you, nor does she want to be spoken to. She will not eat, and she will do anything to keep from throwing up! She lay on the sofa most of the afternoon, and the only thing I could do to help was to supply her with cool washcloths for her face and ice chips to munch on. I felt helpless once again. Finally, she went to bed and was pretty much bedridden for five days. Her body was courageously fighting the chemotherapy drugs, trying to save the cells and it was terrible. I thought of the line in the television movie, *The Temptations,* where one of the group member's mother had cancer, and whenever he visited her and asked how she was doing, she said, "I was doing pretty good until they started curing me!" I could definitely relate to that line of thinking.

Another side effect in the first week was mouth sores. Dr. Hinton and his team had seemed to have seen it all before and could prescribe a drug or treatment for any complication Phyllis had, which was reassuring. He prescribed Diflucan to help with this problem. Plain old ice helped too. Russell knew his mother especially liked the ice from the local Taco Casa, especially when she was dealing with the blisters in her mouth caused by the treatments. He went through the drive-through on the way to visit her and ordered by saying, "My Mom has cancer and she wants just ice—no cola."

I am fortunate to be in a profession where I can adjust my schedule, so I took care of Phyllis most of the time in the beginning of the chemotherapy. But her mother and Caroline helped me out much that first week.

I took the job of making sure she stayed on schedule with her meds. It was a long list, and I seemed to be constantly adding to it. She was a good patient as far as taking her medication, but I could not get her to eat anything of substance. I had the most success with watermelon chunks, but everything she ate went through her quickly because of another side effect of chemotherapy, which is diarrhea. It was a vicious cycle for the first few days.

The first week of chemotherapy treatment had been tough. I sat beside my wife, fighting panic, as I watched her shake uncontrollably, wondering if this was normal before they gave her the Benadryl that stopped it. Getting through that long day was a small victory, but the next five days were horrendous. Dealing with the nausea, diarrhea, weakness, and mouth sores made me wonder how in the heck this was a cure. Again I'd quietly stand in the door of our bedroom where she was resting, watching her chest to make she was breathing. I learned quickly the side effects would be, as her Dad would say, "A hard row to hoe."

First Week as Caregiver

Unable to get any work done at the office, I stayed on my nursing schedule that first week, making sure she took her medication on time. But day by day, she continued to weaken, so on Tuesday, five days after the first treatment, I called Dr. Hinton's office. I was concerned with how weak she was and asked him if this was normal. He told me to bring her in immediately, making me feel guilty that I hadn't called sooner. I had to hold her up as I helped her into the car. When we arrived at Manderson Cancer Center, there was no argument from Phyllis when I parked in the reserved space directly in front of the entrance that was for Manderson Cancer Center patients. The same parking space she had refused to park at a few days earlier pointing out, "Those are for the cancer patients." I wrapped my arm around her waist and almost had to carry her into the Cancer Center's waiting area. I was given her number, and we waited to be called. I could not imagine continuing this for four more months without her being hospitalized.

It was a short wait for the physician. She was given a Decadron shot, a steroid used for many medical conditions, and fluids through her mediport. By that afternoon she was 100% better. I was relieved but felt like a failure that I had not called the doctor sooner. It had been a grim reminder of how serious this battle was, and I wouldn't make that mistake twice.

Stepping into the Ring for Round Two

The next week, Phyllis went in to receive Round Two. I enjoyed thinking of it as rounds in a heavyweight-boxing match with our local hero Deontay Wilder. We had been knocked to the mat last week but had managed to get up before the eight count. We went to our corner, and with the help of Decadron, were able to regroup and continue the fight. I didn't want to think about it being an eighteen-round fight, though. Round Two was expected to be easier with fewer side effects, and this week she would receive only one drug: Herceptin.

It was the same process as the first treatment. Go to the desk, get your number, wait to be called, feel that you shouldn't be there with all the sick folks. This time when they weighed her and took her vitals, we prayed she hadn't lost ten pounds, which would have postponed the treatment. Luckily, she'd only lost nine pounds. Phyllis cheered because she did not want to miss a treatment, and being a woman, was maybe a little happy about losing a few pounds. We took any victory, no matter how small. We headed back to the treatment area, hoping to get a window seat and then settled in for the wait.

HER2 / neu

Round Two was much better. Herceptin, a HER2/neu inhibitor, was part of the three-drug trifecta that Phyllis would receive every third week, but it was also the drug she received at the next two weekly treatments. Taxol, Carboplatin, and Herceptin were week one; Herceptin week two; and Herceptin week three. Then the three-drug cycle started over.

The wonder drug Herceptin has saved hundreds of thousands of lives since Dr. Dennis Slamon, the physician credited most with its development, spent 1988 through 1996 at UCLA Medical Center developing it. I'm always in awe of the intelligent men and women who've dedicated their lives to such noble causes as finding cures for incurable diseases. Dr. Slamon's story is well-documented in the film, *Living Proof,* starring Harry Connick, Jr. It's based on the book by Robert Bazell titled *HER-2: The Making of Herceptin, a Revolutionary Treatment for Breast Cancer.* Phyllis had watched the movie during her chemotherapy, but I wouldn't join her thinking to myself it would be too depressing. But I did watch the movie while doing research for this book, and after seeing it, I wished we had watched it together. I highly recommend the book and movie.

Herceptin increased Phyllis' chances of defeating cancer, and we were playing the odds on this one.

The second treatment was completed at four o'clock that afternoon, and we soon began to call the second and third treatments in each cycle the "easy" ones, if there was such a thing as an easy chemotherapy treatment. The side effects were minimal, and Phyllis could usually function on a normal level, only having to deal with the fatigue.

Round Three

Round Three was much like Round Two—not too bad. We would stay on this schedule throughout the entire duration of chemotherapy treatments. The three-drug cocktail treatment left her completely wiped out, and the second and third were somewhat easier. This allowed her body a slight break from the stress while continuing the fight. There's something comforting about becoming familiar with a pattern—even one so strange and morose as this. All breast cancer treatments are not the same, and some are much more aggressive because of the different types of cancer there are. Even though Phyllis' treatments were bad, compared to what we had researched and had been told by friends who were breast cancer survivors, it could have been much worse, especially if she had required radiation.

Our family was getting into the chemo routine with us, though, and it was evident at Starbucks one day. Caroline and Phyllis were shopping at Midtown in Tuscaloosa and stopped into Starbucks for a pick-me-up of afternoon coffee. When they saw the long line, Caroline suggested saying, "Excuse me, my mother has cancer. Could we please move to front of the line?" Phyllis held her back. She said she felt well enough to wait.

But just before Round Three, something happened that took the wind out of Phyllis' sails. Her hair started falling out.

Chapter 15

LOSING HER HAIR

P hyllis lost a part of her womanhood when her breast was surgically removed, and it was a traumatic event in her view of herself as a woman. Then, two weeks into chemo, something almost equally devastating to her self-image happened. Phyllis' hair started falling out. I remember that it was the twelfth day after chemo began. It first started to fall out as she was brushing it, then it started falling out in clumps in the shower.

I could not have been prouder of how my wife handled this. She said she cried at first, but she is a woman of strong will and resolve. She was determined not to be a victim. Taking matters into her own hands, on September 17, the day before her third chemo treatment, she asked her hairdresser, Ashley

They laughed together and cried together, but most of all, they declared through that act that Phyllis would not be passive.

Martin, to shave her head. They laughed together and cried together, but most of all, they declared through that act that Phyllis would not be passive. She would act, and she would not act alone. Those of us who loved her would support her however we could.

I was expecting a different reaction from Phyllis than she displayed when she lost her hair. I never saw her cry about it. I was expecting much more drama surrounding this event, but as her friend Sharon Gurley shared with her in a very unique way, "You're just going to have to put on your big girl panties and deal with it." And that's what she did. I admired her strength and preparation through this part of the breast cancer treatments because I knew it was a big deal.

Phyllis is a planner and she had prepared for the day her hair would start falling out by going to Birmingham for an emotional day of shopping for a wig. She made the trip without me because it was hard for her to accept the fact that I would be seeing her without hair. She took her mother with her instead for a second opinion and to ease her mother into the realization that her daughter was going to lose her hair. Phyllis made it a fun outing for her mother Doris and even got her to try on one! They found one that matched her own hair almost perfectly. It was amazing! It wasn't cheap, but it was beautiful and worth every dollar of the five hundred it cost.

I was prepared for her hair loss, and I had steeled myself against all the negative fallout from a wife who had lost her hair. I was expecting many tears, but they never came, at least not in my presence. I was prepared for any misdirected anger that might come my way, but it never materialized. Every day, she simply put on a nice wig and went about her business. I was proud to be the husband of such a courageous woman. I made an effort to see her without the wigs or caps or scarves. She needed to know it was just me, the guy that had been with her since they were teenagers and to understand I was okay with it. Like Bruno Mars said in his song, "I love you just the way you are."

Most of the people Phyllis came in contact with never knew she was wearing a wig because it looked so much like her original hair color and style and were shocked when they discovered it was a wig. And she was in contact with a lot of people! During her year of chemotherapy treatments, she was the Tuscaloosa Association of Realtors Incoming President and was in charge of securing a guest speaker for the monthly meetings of Realtors in the Association. At these meetings, she stood in front of two hundred plus colleagues and provided information pertinent to our local and national industry. After she had served her year as Incoming President, she became the President of the Tuscaloosa Association of Realtors, and during her first speech, she never once mentioned that she had been taking chemotherapy for the last few months. Many had no idea she had had breast cancer or that she was wearing a wig. She was truly Super Woman the entire time that sought no pity.

When her hair first started falling out, she was shy about me seeing her without her wig, but I assured her time and again that I thought she was as beautiful as ever and she was. Initially, she wore a scarf or cap around me, but she finally loosened up and allowed me to see her bald. She had a pretty, round head and I became fond of that bare head. I wasn't worried about her hair. I only wanted her to be cured of breast cancer and live forever.

Only those of us in her immediate family were allowed to see her go "commando," as we called it. We would all rub her head for luck. It was like a pregnant woman when folks just wanted to touch her belly or like a gazing ball in a garden. Our granddaughters Olivia and Marlys couldn't get enough of it. Her bald head didn't bother them one bit because they loved "Gigi" no matter what. I'll never forget how Olivia, at five years old, told someone that her Gigi had "a little cancer." Adorable. Marlys, three at the time, always searched for and found the Mediport on her Gigi's chest and would rub it as she fell to sleep. After it was removed when Phyllis had completed all treatments, Marlys still felt for it.

That wig, vital as it was, seemed to have a mind of its own. On more than one occasion I walked into our bathroom and caught a glimpse of what I thought was a head on the counter, and it scared the you-know-what out of me! It was like the Elf on the Shelf. I never knew where it would pop up. Sometimes it looked like a head lying in our bathtub but it was only her spare, drying off after she'd washed it. Phyllis found this amusing, and I'm not sure but I think she derived much pleasure from surprising me in this manner. Whatever it took to get her smiling!

Phyllis was baking one afternoon and hurriedly removed the dish from the oven. The dish was baking at four hundred degrees, and she tried to grab it as soon as she opened the oven door. The heat did a number on the wig, singeing it and requiring an additional trip to Ashley, the hairdresser, for a trim. Phyllis advised many women to be careful taking anything out of a four hundred-degree oven with a wig on!

Having to wear a wig was traumatic enough, but the day Phyllis noticed her eyelashes and eyebrows were falling out was intense. She walked by me announcing in colorful language, "Now my &$!# eyebrows and eyelashes are falling out!" We had known that was a possibility, but they had hung on well into the chemo treatments and she was happy for that little victory. Losing those was the straw that broke the camel's back. Having no choice, she eventually accepted it but still complains about it to this day.

Breast cancer wouldn't even let her keep her eyebrows and eyelashes.

Chapter 16

CHEMOTHERAPY ROUTINE

A s we got into the chemotherapy routine, Phyllis decided to make the best of her time while being confined to her chemotherapy recliner. She never watched the television at the Cancer Center but instead spent most of her time setting appointments for her real estate business, posting pictures on social media of her adventure, making telephone calls, texting me to-do lists, praying, and napping.

As uncomfortable as it was, Phyllis accepted the gift of slowing down and really thinking about how precious life is. Much good came from her downtime. It was good for our relationship because I was taking the time to sit with her and talk. It is easy to focus on real life issues while sitting with your loved one while she's taking chemotherapy.

We were fortunate that we lived and worked a couple of miles from Manderson Cancer Center. As I became more comfortable with the chemotherapy routine, I was able to take Phyllis to the Cancer Center and make sure she was set up, and then I would go to the office or go show property. She preferred that I be out working.

So, while I didn't spend every minute with Phyllis at her treatments, I did try to make an appearance at every one. I'd take her a nice lunch, at least, and she was always glad to see me. Sometimes I brought Krispy Kreme doughnuts or Edgar's Red Velvet Cheesecake Brownies that the nurses helped devour! That got us both some brownie points.

Support from Friends

There was no danger of her being alone for any length of time anyway. She had an outpouring of love from friends and family who wanted to come and sit with her during her treatments. Since I was the unofficial gate keeper, I laughed and told them, "I'll check our schedule and put you on standby in case there's a cancellation!" Phyllis used this time to reconnect with old acquaintances and build new relationships. She worked out her own friend-sitting schedule without any assistance from me.

One of the most pleasant surprises we had during this adventure was the genuine empathy that was directed Phyllis' way. Both women and men would sincerely take the time to seek her out through emails, texts, letters, cards, and face-to-face conversations. It was amazing and somewhat humbling to have that much love directed your way.

The women seemed to have the most empathy because they could certainly imagine the possibility of being in the same situation. They feared that they too might be diagnosed with breast cancer someday and have to have a single or double mastectomy, or they feared that they too might someday lose their hair during chemotherapy. They feared that it would be them feeling unattractive. They feared the uncertainty of breast cancer, and they feared the very real possibility of death.

Several breast cancer survivors sought her out to share their experience and to give her advice of how to handle it. Some would pray with her, and we accepted all prayers. Jean Minges was one such breast cancer survivor. She was so generous with her time and prayers for Phyllis. Jean is a fellow Realtor with another real estate company in Tuscaloosa and didn't

That sincere act touched me greatly and still brings tears to my eyes whenever I remember how true a moment that was.

let the competitive nature of our business interfere with her sharing. She was very honest and would answer any question Phyllis had. I discovered Jean's Godly character when she called Phyllis early on and asked if she could come by our home and visit. I was busy, giving them their privacy, when I looked into our den and saw Jean was holding Phyllis' hand, praying for her healing. That sincere act touched me greatly and still brings tears to my eyes whenever I remember how true a moment that was. Jean sat with Phyllis on several occasions at the Cancer Center and was very honest in sharing her experiences, both good and bad. I didn't worry about Phyllis one bit while Jean was with her.

Another dear friend who was so honest and open about her experience was Kim Wolbach. Kim is also a Realtor with yet another real estate company in Tuscaloosa and a breast cancer survivor too. Kim also sat with Phyllis during chemotherapy and led her, step by step, through each process, candidly sharing her experience as only Kim can. She would get on a roll and suddenly stop and say, "I can't believe I just said that in front of Ken!" I didn't mind, and it didn't embarrass me because I wanted to be part of the conversation so I would know what to expect too. I became one of the girls! I first learned about tattooed areolas and nipples from Kim! She was my comic relief.

Both of these ladies shared their experience with reconstructive surgery, and it helped Phyllis get her mind off the present situation and begin thinking about future possibilities. Jean told Phyllis, "reconstructive surgery won't create centerfold breasts, but you will be surprised at what a plastic surgeon can do." She wasn't trying to be humorous, but I thought that funny!

Correspondence

One of the activities that helped Phyllis pass the time while taking chemotherapy was reading the cards, letters, and emails from her many friends. People would take the time from their busy schedules, and while thinking about Phyllis, write her a note. It was humbling to feel that much love.

Phyllis at first hoped to keep her diagnosis a secret because she said, "cancer is really bad for public relations." She finally decided that it would be impossible to keep this news private, so she sent the following email to all those that worked with RE/MAX Premiere Group.

Subject: Personal News
Thursday, July 31, 2014

Many of us have worked together and been friends for twenty years. You feel like family, so I want to share some news with you before you hear it from someone else.

I have recently been diagnosed with breast cancer. Because I naively thought I would have the surgery and be back at work in a couple of days, I had hoped to remain private. But unfortunately, Dr. David Hinton recommends aggressive chemotherapy and possibly radiation later. I won't be able to keep those side effects secret. My surgery is scheduled for Tuesday. David will begin my treatments about three weeks following.

This news of course has been overwhelming but I am so blessed with support of my family and friends. Ken, as always, is my rock.

Another great blessing has been Iris and David Hinton helping me navigate through this quickly and David's immediate availability any time I have a question.

I plan to continue working and living my life as normally as I can. None of my meetings or trips have been cancelled. I will make adjustments I'm sure but cancer won't be my career. And the silver lining is I'll get to try a new hairstyle! Maybe a sassy redhead!

I appreciate all of you.

Minutes later the responses started, and here is the first:

I am so sorry to hear this Phyllis. I love you to death and have the utmost respect for you as a friend and as a Boss/Business associate, so you know that if there is anything I can do to help you and Ken I will do it.

Your Friend,

Doug

I would love to be your driver. I'd be honored to spend a little more time with you.

Vanessa

My heart is heavy with this news and I will keep sweet Phyllis in my prayers. She's strong and I know she's going to do great!

Teresa

Watch what you wish for, those girls I have been around that are redheads are really strange creatures! Take care and know that you are being lifted up.

James (married to a redhead)

Our family will be lifting you up in prayer. David wrote:
I will lift up my eyes to the hills from whence cometh my help.
My help cometh from the Lord. The Lord who made heaven and
Earth. He said he will not suffer my foot to be moved the Lord
which keepeth thee, he will not slumber nor sleep. Sometimes when
we get in the midst of a storm we need to be reminded our lifeguard
walks on water!
Pam

Pam had just quoted Phyllis' favorite verse! Here's what Phyllis wrote back:

Pam, Psalms 121 is my favorite scripture because it was
Daddy's favorite. He scribbled it down for me once when I was in
a difficult period. Tuesday morning after I learned I would need
chemo, that very scripture was on my verse of the day flip calendar
by my coffee pot. I thought Daddy had sent an angel to remind me
to not be afraid. And then he did again through your email. I don't
believe those were coincidences.
Phyllis

Phyllis received literally hundreds of emails and cards in the days and weeks to come. One from our sixteen-year-old neighbor, Quinn Edmonds, stood out. Quinn is a young man with an old soul. He's the neighborhood lawn care specialist and has been running his lawn care business (with employees) since he was fourteen. Often, we would come home from chemotherapy to find Quinn voluntarily cutting our lawn. He had recently lost his close grandfather unexpectedly and quickly to cancer. Here is his heart-felt letter written at age sixteen.

11/6/14

Mrs. Phyllis,

Listed below are a few Bible verses that I shared with my grandfather. They gave him comfort and reassurance in the darkest and hardest days of his battle with cancer. I hope you will be able to find a similar comfort in them.

"Be strong and courageous. Do not be afraid or terrified because of them, for the Lord your God goes with you! He will never leave you nor forsake you." Deuteronomy 31:6

"For I know the plans I have for you, declares the Lord. Plans to prosper you and not to harm you. Plans to give you a hope and a future. Then you will come to me, and I will listen to you. You will seek me and find me when you seek me with all your heart. Jeremiah 29: 11-13

"Even youths grow tired and weary and young men stumble and fall; but those who hope in the Lord will renew their strength. They will soar on wings like eagles; they will run and not grow weary, they will walk and not be faint." Isaiah 40: 30-31

These verses are our prayer for you as you continue this fight. The Lord loves you and though we do not always understand his reasons and his ways, his ways are higher than ours. We are praying for you and love you dearly.

-Quinn Edmonds

Reading notes like these would make Phyllis very introspective, but even on chemotherapy days, she continued working. Once while nurse Tammy was starting the infusion, she overheard Phyllis talking to a client on the phone as if she were sitting in her real estate office. Tammy commented, "They have no idea you're sitting here getting a chemo treatment!"

Phyllis always was dressed to the nines when she went to take her treatments. She smiled and hid her pain. I saw the true effects when we were alone, though, and it will break your spirit if you let it. I had made up my mind early on that there was no way it would break my spirit, and I would fight with her. I had to learn how to help, and it was always the little things I did that made a difference with her. She made the best of a bad situation, but there really is no way to sugarcoat chemotherapy.

We still dreaded that first treatment of the cycle when the three chemotherapy drugs were given. It led to excessive pain and suffering every single time.

Our New Normal

Over the course of our marriage, Phyllis and I have been known to, let's just say, express our opinions fervently to each other. We only had one argument the entire time she was dealing with breast cancer, and that was when I tried, unsuccessfully, to get her to take it easy. It was frustrating for me to see her push herself to needless limits, but as frustrated as I was, she was more frustrated at the limitations cancer was putting on her. She refused to let me limit her even further.

I'll never forget how Phyllis insisted on going to a women's Christian conference at Church of the Highlands in Birmingham, Alabama, with Caroline and Mary Hughes, the day after taking the second three-drug combo in the cycle. She was feeling stronger after the last two weekly treatments of Herceptin and had apparently forgotten what the first treatment of the cycle felt like. That trip did not work out as planned. She began feeling the side effects and had to come home and go to bed. Two days later, though, and feeling better, she headed to Mobile, Alabama, for the Alabama Association of Realtors annual convention for a three-day event. The next week she accompanied me to the RE/MAX Dixie Region Broker/Owner Bestfest Convention in Biloxi, Mississippi. At least there I was able to care for her, and the only problem we had was walking through the casino getting to our conference hall. Her wig absorbed the stale cigarette smoke and this displeased her greatly!

Throughout that year of chemotherapy, I tried in vain to get Phyllis to slow down and take it easy. But it was like what her Daddy said once about a family member who was trying to get him to slow down a little with his gardening: "They're just wasting good air telling me to quit." Most of the time I felt I was wasting good air. She is strong-willed and determined to not be a victim, but sometimes that got her into trouble.

Like the time Phyllis had listed a nice home on Lake Tuscaloosa in the Stone Harbour Subdivision in Northport, Alabama. The owners were moving due to a job transfer to Mississippi. It was a lakefront property but access to the lake was limited because of the steep terrain. This did not stop Phyllis from taking pictures of the waterfront. She was in the middle of chemotherapy treatments, weak but not believing it.

She made her way down the steep bank and took several great pictures of the water with her iPhone, believing that these pictures would be what sold the house. So far, so good. But getting back to the top was a different story. It was hot and humid of course, being in Alabama, and she had to literally pull herself to the top by holding onto small bushes and the big oak tree roots on the side of the bluff. Sweat was pouring out from under her wig, and she was close to fainting when she finally made it to the top where she immediately laid down in the yard, realizing she had overestimated her present abilities. She drove herself home and went straight to bed.

That evening when she told me about her adventure that day, I could only shake my head in disbelief. Phyllis said, "I got those pictures though!" Yes, she did and she did it in heels! I could only reason it was due to Chemo Brain. Whenever she did something hard to defend, instead of pleading ignorance she simply blamed it on chemo brain.

One other situation she got both of us into was when she became a firebug.

Our RE/MAX office is about one mile from our house, which was definitely convenient for me when Phyllis was home recuperating. I could keep a check on her by quickly running home to make sure she was okay.

Our backyard backs up to the street that leads in to our subdivision. Planted against the brick wall that separates us from the street is a privacy hedge of Little Gem Magnolias and Holly trees that were beginning to make a nice blind. As I was making my way home to check on Phyllis and approaching the spot where I could see our backyard, I saw smoke. Lots of smoke! I accelerated, got to the house fast, and ran into the backyard through the iron gate to find Phyllis fighting a grass fire!

She informed me she had wanted to get a little exercise outside and was picking up the dead limbs and sticks. (Her heart rate was certainly accelerated, as was mine!) She had then decided to burn them in the copper fire pit, but it is usually dry in the fall in Tuscaloosa and it was dry as a bone that day.

She was in a panic and had tried everything to put out the fire that was getting out of control. Everything except the garden hose because she could not get it hooked up. Phyllis fought the fire with green limbs broken off the Little Gems, and she pulled the rug on the patio over the blaze, only to catch it on fire too. She even used her little cap that covered her pretty bald head to fight the flames.

I quickly helped her get it under control by connecting the difficult garden hose. I didn't get mad and tell her she was crazy or ask her, "What were you thinking?" I felt for her because she was embarrassed that she had burned a large portion of our backyard lawn, but I hurt for her the most because she seemed defeated. In her mind, she was exposed without something covering her head outside of the house. We eventually laughed about it, which was better than crying.

We decided two things that day. One: God was directing me home that day at the perfect time. We had put out fires all our married life, so this was no big deal. And two: always make sure the garden hose is connected and turned on before burning sticks.

I also told her the grass would grow back like her hair. Someday.

Chapter 17

KEEPING TRADITIONS

Traditions are important to me and my family, so during Phyllis' battle with breast cancer, it was important to me to make sure everyone in our clan followed and observed our traditions as best we could.

Many of our traditions center around the kitchen and dining room table. I can think of worse things than gathering all your family around a table to say a prayer of thanks and just enjoy each other's company. This was never more true than during Thanksgiving 2014.

Thanksgiving 2014

Breast cancer treatment does not take time off for the holidays. Phyllis' chemotherapy treatment was scheduled for November 26, which was the day before Thanksgiving. It was number five of Round One (the big bad one), where she received the three drugs and number thirteen treatment overall. We knew that she would need to recuperate after that treatment, and by now the drugs were taking their toll. She was struggling with her energy level.

We take turns hosting with our extended families, and the year of Phyllis' chemotherapy was our year to host my extended family. I thought we had the best excuse in the world to skip our turn, but Phyllis decided we'd host anyway.

Breast cancer treatment does not take time off for the holidays.

We'd just do it on the twenty-sixth, the day before Thanksgiving. She'd just have to leave in the early afternoon for her chemotherapy treatment. Everyone objected at first, saying, "Surely she'll be too tired and not feel like entertaining," but we held our ground. And I know they were secretly pleased that we would keep the Thanksgiving tradition going. There'd be plenty of people to help share the cooking duties. But the family faced a dilemma. Who would cook the chicken and dressing? Phyllis was always in charge of making her famous chicken and dressing, and her chicken and dressing is excellent. It's a meal in itself.

Now, for you northerners, there's a big difference between *dressing* and *stuffing*. Phyllis' chicken and dressing is moist, rich with butter, and real broth from a baked roasting hen. One reason Phyllis agreed to carry on the Thanksgiving tradition at our home is that I offered to help her make it. My job was to make the cornbread, cook the hen, and then debone it. That's right! I stepped up, guys! Her job would be to put it all together once I had my part finished. I had confidence it would be edible because chicken and dressing begins with good cornbread, and I make excellent cornbread. However, we were both a little concerned because she doesn't have a recipe—she just tastes as she goes and adjusts as needed. She gets in the Goldie Locks tasting zone and gets it just right! Chemotherapy had ruined her taste buds, so the taste-testing would fall on me. I have to admit I was a little apprehensive about that duty.

It was Thanksgiving Eve Eve and time for me to get started. As stated earlier, cornbread is a main ingredient in southern chicken and dressing, and my cornbread has a story all its own. Phyllis' dad, Johnny, and I grew the corn that our cornmeal was made from. See, Johnny was a master gardener, and he did not become one by going to classes. It was his passion and he did it well, so I wanted to learn as much about gardening from him as possible. I had a farm a few miles from Johnny's house that grew excellent vegetables, and for a few of his last years, we gardened together. He taught me to plant enough for everyone in our extended family. Planting is fun, but the hard work of harvesting and preserving is a different story.

I planted a sweet corn called Mirai, and I was proud when Johnny said it was the best he had ever had, which was saying a lot—getting a compliment out of him was not easy. But my favorite gardening project with him was the acre of White Moseby corn we planted for the specific use of making cornmeal to make our cornbread. I thought Johnny's cornbread was the best. It had a coarse texture that was different from any other I had tried.

The White Moseby corn patch was a huge success! Like everything else in my life, I tried to make it a family project, so that included getting the men involved. Russell helped with thinning the corn once it grew to about eight inches, then he and A. J. helped their eighty-year-old grandfather gather the corn once it had dried enough on the stalk. I remember them saying Johnny outworked them both. Once the dry corn was gathered, it was time to shuck the corn and shell it. Shelling the corn was fun because Johnny had an ancient corn sheller that simply required you to put the dried ear of corn in and turn the metal crank. Out one exit popped the clean corncob, and the other side emptied the white dried corn.

Johnny and I then took several fifty-pound bags of shelled corn to Mr. Simmons' in Duncanville, Alabama, to have him grind our corn into cornmeal. We chose him because Johnny said he had a nice, clean electric mill in his shop, and he liked his work. That day we ground sixty gallon bags of cornmeal for us to keep, and Mr. Simmons wanted ten bags as payment for his services.

I was proud that day. There is no more honest work than planting a seed, taking care of something as it grows, and then enjoying the fruits of your labor. Nothing tastes as good as food grown in your own garden.

> *There is no more honest work than planting a seed, taking care of something as it grows, and then enjoying the fruits of your labor.*

As I was making the cornbread for Thanksgiving that year, I was especially mindful of Johnny. He had a profound influence on mine and Phyllis' life with his work ethic and the sacrifices he made for his family. She said she was glad he didn't have to see her suffer through breast cancer because she knew it would hurt him so.

I made three pones (translation: pans) of cornbread that night. Each batch had one teaspoon of baking powder, one teaspoon of salt, two tablespoons of sugar, two eggs, a pinch of baking soda, around four cups of our cornmeal, and enough buttermilk to make it easy to pour. I heated the oven to four hundred and thirty degrees and put my heirloom iron skillets into the oven. Once they were hot enough, I put the butter in the iron skillets and when the butter was sizzling, in went the mixture. You know you're doing it right when the mixture starts cooking as soon as it hits the hot iron. Twenty to thirty minutes later, the basic ingredient for chicken and dressing was done. It came from a seed I had planted with Phyllis' daddy, Johnny. I knew she liked that cornbread mainly because her father had a hand in it. The best traditions are usually the simplest ones that remind us of loved ones that have already gone on.

While the oven was hot, I placed the roasting hen in the oven with salt, pepper, butter, and plenty of water to make the broth. The house smelled like the home of our childhoods and reminded Phyllis and me of simpler times with our brothers and sisters. After a couple hours of slow-cooking that hen, we took it out of the oven and allowed it to cool. I set about deboning the chicken and straining the broth, then packed it up and put it in the refrigerator.

The next morning, I crumbled the bread just like Phyllis told me to—careful not to squeeze it together or it would be gummy. I lined up all the necessary ingredients on the kitchen counter, waiting for her input. Chicken broth, cream of chicken soup, salt, pepper, sage (but not too much), and the shredded baked hen went into the big crumbled pan of cornbread. I was paying close attention when she held up a spoon full of the mixture and asked, "Does it have enough sage?" It was the moment of truth. I fearlessly tasted and informed her that I tasted no sage. She said, "Good. It's easier to add than take away." We finally got it right, or so I hoped, and we had fun sharing the moment.

The chicken and dressing was a huge success and so was our Thanksgiving celebration, even in the year of breast cancer. The meal was a feast with my sister Rita bringing her dill pickle deviled eggs, my brother, Ronnie, and his seven-layer salad, the nieces bringing their buttermilk pie, mashed potatoes, and green beans. Before we began eating, I asked for God's blessings on the meal while thanking him for carrying us through the last few months. I was emotional, and the granddaughters wondered why Poppy was crying. I was not alone with my tears. There wasn't a dry eye in my house. We were fighting hard to keep some sort of normalcy in our loved ones' lives.

Phyllis had to leave for her chemotherapy treatment at two thirty. I stayed home with my family and for cleanup duty. We all pitched in, and it didn't take long. I even managed to toss a wooden spoon in the dishwater while my niece Robin was washing dishes. For some reason, this makes her gag, and I love making her do it. It's tradition! It was the best Thanksgiving ever, and I was thankful my family was still intact.

A Chemo Christmas

I have a reputation: I complain too much at Christmas. Getting caught up in my required duties of the holiday can bring out the Scrooge in me. But this breast cancer Christmas I resolved to be different. I would be on my best behavior. Phyllis had always done most of the shopping, decorating the tree, cooking and buying gifts, so my goal in 2014 was to take on as much of that load as possible to make it easier for her. She had been through a rough year, to say the least, so it was time to keep my Scrooge tendencies at bay.

We were so happy that the exhausting treatments were winding down. They had taken their toll on her body. She was frustrated with the fatigue and was certainly tired of the chemotherapy routine. She'd made it through a major holiday with Thanksgiving, and now she had another chemo appointment scheduled for Christmas Eve. It was a strange way to mark the calendar. I still wished I could have suffered through it for her.

I had decided it was certainly her year for a big gift from me, and it needed to be special. One that she would remember for the rest of our lives. After searching online for ideas and coming up empty, I stopped by Fincher and Ozment, a local upscale jewelry store. They were quick to wait on me. A middle-aged man walking in at Christmas must be a good prospect for a commissioned salesperson.

Usually I go into a store and decide what gift to buy fairly quickly, but this gift required more thoughtful deliberation. There were many baubles to choose from, and the saleslady was good at her job. We looked at several diamonds in many settings, but I saw nothing that I thought looked like Phyllis. I explained to the saleslady that my wife was fighting breast cancer and asked if she had any gemstones that were pink, thinking that might work while acknowledging breast cancer awareness.

"Are you familiar with Morganite?" she asked.

I wasn't, so she gave me a quick lesson and informed me the gemstone Beryl, formed in several colors with the most recognizable one being the emerald. The pink color of Beryl is called Morganite. After seeing the gemstone, I thought it would be perfect. Now to find the perfect setting.

She presented several pieces that were petite.

"This is the year to go gaudy!" I said.

She brought out a lovely, big Morganite gemstone ring surrounded by diamond clusters. It was pricey but it was perfect for the occasion, so I bought it! Looking back, maybe I needed to feel some pain too! I could hardly wait to give the ring to her, but I had to make myself wait until Christmas morning.

Phyllis had chemotherapy treatment number seventeen on Christmas Eve morning. She took the nurses who'd helped her along her road a few edible gifts from the bakery. They adored her and her positive attitude.

On Christmas Eve, I was almost as excited as little Olivia and Marlys. Almost. Children getting presents does make Christmas exciting.

Our Christmas celebration began on Christmas Eve with my family gathering at our house. We used this time to wind down and to start focusing on the reason for the season. We read the story of Jesus' birth. We opened the traditional Christmas Eve gifts from Phyllis: new pajamas for everyone except me. I got a new t-shirt. Phyllis felt everyone should have new pajamas for the Christmas morning snapshots.

Russell and Caroline left with their families, and they celebrated Christmas morning at their own homes with their personal gifts. The granddaughters got their Santa gifts when they awoke early Christmas morning, but then they quickly headed for Poppy and Gigi's for more gifts and breakfast. Caroline's family arrived around 8:00 a.m. and even Russell and Amanda made it on time, which was a Christmas miracle in itself!

After everyone arrived, we gathered in the den looking fine in our new pajamas. We tried to make it last as long as possible by each getting only one gift at a time, but we soon gave way to the chaos. The little girls got toys and books, the big girls got clothes and gift cards, and the men got gun stuff and tools. There were M&M's and gum in the stockings (it's tradition), and I dropped folding money in to make sure they all wouldn't be broke.

After everyone else had opened their presents, we were ready for Phyllis to open her gifts. Like her Daddy, Phyllis enjoys watching others open their gifts more than opening her own. She also feels the need to explain that the gifts she gave could be exchanged if it doesn't fit or if they prefer another color or to tell the story of what she went through to get that present here on time. I guess that's tradition too.

She finally started opening her gifts, and being pretty crafty, she opened the large boxes first and saved the little box from me for last. Carefully unwrapping the little box, she stole a quick look at me. Her brown eyes got big, and they filled with tears along with the rest of us.

"It's pink!" she said, immediately recognizing the significance of the color.

I was emotional, the kids were emotional, and above all else, Phyllis was happy. Best Christmas ever! Not because I spent too much money, but because we all knew how blessed we were to be together. Our faith as a family was strong, and Phyllis' suffering had made us stronger.

> *Our faith as a family was strong, and Phyllis' suffering had made us stronger.*

As the wave of emotions finally subsided, we all agreed it was time for breakfast. Opening gifts is merely the appetizer for our traditional breakfast starring Phyllis' homemade biscuits. I headed to the kitchen, eager to be doing something that would dry my eyes, and brought out the big iron skillet again. I filled it with Tennessee Pride breakfast sausage because sausage drippings make the best sawmill gravy. I know, not healthy, but it's tradition! Phyllis started kneading the dough for her delicious biscuits. She put two iron skillets in the oven to warm. When the dough and the pans were ready, she placed the biscuits close together, stole a few spoonsful of sausage drippings from my pan to brush their tops, and popped them in the oven.

I made the sawmill gravy, checking with Phyllis occasionally to make sure I was doing it right. We'd eat the sawmill gravy with biscuits or eggs.

When we finished cooking, and it was ready to eat, we gathered around the big oak dinner table and I asked God's blessings on the meal and the hands that prepared it. I didn't forget the true meaning of Christmas and thanked Him for sending his Son, the Baby Jesus. I also didn't forget to offer a special thank-you for his healing power and his mercy that allowed us all to be together. We'd also made our once-a-year Christmas breakfast tradition of chocolate gravy. It's a thin chocolate concoction that you pour over your hot biscuits for dessert. So of course, we all ate too much. It's tradition!

Florida

The Olive family has been going to the Florida Gulf Coast for as long as our kids can remember. Phyllis and I started over forty years ago when we went to Fort Walton Beach for our honeymoon. It was the first time I had seen the ocean and the sugar white sands of the Gulf of Mexico. Maybe it was the honeymoon, but I immediately fell in love with the place.

Over the years we somehow migrated east along the coast to Destin and discovered the fishing village that included the Kelly Docks where scenes from the movie Jaws were filmed. Along the docks was a restaurant called Capt'n Dave's where I ate my first crab claws, fried to perfection and big as two fingers. Destin is where we first took our kids and introduced them to the beach. We found Dewey Destin's on the old docks and had their stuffed shrimp while sitting on the old wooden pier, and the Back Porch that has the best fish baskets and shrimp po'boys.

Before long we began renting houses along the beach so we could have plenty of room for the kids' friends who always seemed to be free the week we went. The houses suited us well because with a kitchen, I could cook some of our meals. After a few years we tried San Destin, farther east still, where we discovered resort living at San Destin Beach Resort. It had great shops, live music, golf, and of course the beach with its fifty dollar-per-day umbrellas. And then we found Seaside, Florida. Seaside was a dream that developer Robert Davis somehow made come true. It's the place we now measure every other place against and where we vacation every year now. Each time we visit Modica's Market to enjoy the folk singing and shop for staples for the kitchen, Sun Dog Books, and The Roof Deck Bar at Bud and Allie's for the crab cakes at sunset.

One of our most memorable trips to Seaside was in February 2015, but not for reasons you might expect. Phyllis was finished with the eighteen chemotherapy treatments with only her every-third-week of Herceptin required, but she was still trying to gather her strength back. I had some writing I wanted to do, so I rented a little two-bedroom cottage in Seaside called Dreamsicle that was hidden behind the larger houses on Tupelo Street. You could hardly see it from the street, but a wooden arbor showed the way to a natural sandy path that led to the little yellow cottage. The first thing I saw when I arrived was the two red bicycles parked at the steps of the front porch where a wooden swing swayed in the breeze. It was quaint with a little kitchen—perfect for what I had in mind. We'd rented the place for two weeks and the first week would be mine. I wrote in the mornings, put a jacket on, and read all afternoon in the sun, then ate fresh seafood in the evenings. I even went to the theater and watched the movie called *The Kingsman* one afternoon. It was good to be alone and think.

After I had enjoyed my sabbatical for the week, Russell, Amanda and their dogs came down for a couple of days, so I left them a stocked refrigerator and headed back home. On Monday it was Phyllis,

Caroline, Olivia, and Marlys' turn, and when they arrived they found the refrigerator empty. They hit Seaside and the shops like Hurricane Katrina and stayed the remainder of the week enjoying life.

We'd been through a lot as a family, and that trip was a big part of the healing process for me. I was able to relax after months of being a caregiver and just focus on the future—a future full of hope and new possibilities. I rested knowing Phyllis had made it through the storm of breast cancer and chemotherapy.

Chapter 18
WHAT WILL I DO
IF SHE DIES?

When we married at the young age of seventeen and eighteen, Phyllis and I said those sacred words "'til death do us part," and I meant them. Like every young couple in love, we both thought that the death date was quite a way off. When Phyllis got her diagnosis, I refused to consider the possibility of her dying. Initially, I would not allow myself to even go there with that thought. Every time the thought surfaced, I pushed it down deep into one of those convolutions in my brain. It's still tough for me to write the words that form the sentence that asks the question, "What if Phyllis dies?" My mother, JoAnn, would always say, "Don't speak it into existence!" I guess that's one thing she said to me that stuck.

Besides, I'd been raised to believe what Jesus taught: we're not meant to worry. God will take care of us if we will only have faith, but cancer had a way of changing my thought patterns and jarred me into facing the facts. And with that, my faith may have waivered a bit. When Phyllis was lying in bed the entire week after receiving her first chemotherapy treatment, she and I both wondered how anyone could live through it.

But the fact is, denying the possibility that she could die meant taking Phyllis for granted. I had lost all sense of control of life as I knew it the moment Phyllis said, "It's breast cancer!" But I wondered, had I ever had it to begin with? Are we ever sure our loved one will make it through another day? The answer to that is no, I can't be sure. And this realization made me treasure each day of our journey together. That's why I doubled down to support her both physically and emotionally.

> *I had lost all sense of control of life as I knew it the moment Phyllis said, "It's breast cancer!"*

We'd lost both our fathers recently, so death was very real to us. My dad, Jim, had a long, slow decline, and I was blessed to have a good, clear conversation with him twenty minutes before he died. My mother and brother had taken care of his daily physical needs, and I did everything in my power to make his life worry-free. I was holding his hand as he passed away on my son's birthday. It was the greatest moment I ever had with him.

As I've mentioned, Phyllis' dad, Johnny, gardened every day possible. As we began to anticipate his leaving this world, we decided to support him, encouraging him and making sure he had the supplies needed to make his garden grow. The most treasured memories I have with him are when we were on my farm and he was answering all my questions about growing vegetables. I believe he died knowing I could carry on and grow a garden if need-be to keep his daughter and grandbabies fed.

So, Phyllis and I knew what death looked like, and we knew what a large hole was left in the hearts of the survivors. When our fathers died, it was made easier knowing how respected they were among their friends and families. We'd always had to share our dads with others, and we knew they were both in heaven. The year of Phyllis' breast cancer and chemotherapy brought

So, Phyllis and I knew what death looked like, and we knew what a large hole was left in the hearts of the survivors.

home to me how loved and respected she was, too, and that was a blessing I could hold on to.

However, breast cancer did make us both look at the larger picture and ask ourselves what kind of legacy we would leave behind when we left this earth. Turns out, thinking of legacies and dying made me want to be a better person. It got me to thinking about the meaning of my life and what I could do to make a difference in life instead of death. I have to admit that when I'm gone, I would like to be remembered fondly for the good things I accomplished, and hopefully everyone will forget the bad things I did. When I started thinking along these lines I saw life in a different light. I believe you will always be remembered by how you go about your daily life and what you will do when no one is looking. You will be most remembered by those closest to you, which is family and friends, but sometimes I treated them worse than anyone. This life-changing event caused me to be more respectful of Phyllis and my family's feelings and opinions.

Now I know I can't be a productive man, as God intended, by waking every morning thinking of dying. When you or someone you love has breast cancer, that's easier said than done. Dr. Hinton said that patients would figuratively get in a fetal position or they would hit the diagnosis head on and fight for life. I know Phyllis initially wondered if her time on earth was short because of this disease, and I have to admit it popped up in my mind, too, but I fought the thoughts of her dying every time. But this did make me consider that life is short, and we should be all that we can be. I made a conscious effort to be more in tune with my purpose here.

What will we leave behind? Zig Zeigler once told a joke of two men at the funeral home paying their last respects to their wealthy friend. One asks the other "How much money did he leave?" and the other man replied, "Why, he left it all." It's never about the money, so why do we spend our lives focused on money and not doing good?

The people that have gone on, and that I remember the most, are my mother and father. They were so good to me, and I knew they loved me. Never doubted it. They both lived a holy life and practiced what they preached. I remember Johnny for his hard work and generosity to others and how he never wanted any acknowledgements for his gifts and never boasted that he gave anyone anything. I remember friends like Jimmy Kuykendall and Jackie Kuykendall as friends I could always count on. The people that had an impact on my life were simple folks that were good to my family and me. They didn't judge me or think themselves better than me.

Phyllis and I had talked throughout our marriage about leaving a good legacy behind and what that meant to us as a couple and as individuals. This was especially true at this point in our lives. We talked about the folks in our lives we respected. They always seemed to be just simple people, kind and thoughtful to those around them. We made an effort to be kind and generous to those around us because sometimes it does take a strong effort. In my position as a broker and owner of a real estate company with many people counting on me to make the right decisions, I realize I have a direct influence on them and their family's lives as well. I pray that my influence is always positive on all parties.

The urgency of breast cancer had given me the courage to begin writing a first book at the age of fifty-seven. What better way to be remembered than by writing encouraging words to men and women after a breast cancer diagnosis—one of the lowest and most vulnerable points in their lives? Time will only tell.

So, yes, I did give thought to the possibility that breast cancer could kill my wife. We faced that fact like we did everything else in this adventure: we tried to make lemonade out of life's lemons and grow as Christians. Considering death forced me to consider living a more generous life to those around me.

Would I have done anything differently had I known for a fact that breast cancer would take Phyllis' life? Yes, one thing: I would have taken her anywhere she wanted to go. She loves to travel! So, I'm working on that now, believe me. When she mentions a place she wants to visit, I try to be energetic and pack a bag, and we're off! I must admit she has more energy than me when it comes to traveling, but I'm doing better.

Chapter 19

COULD WE LIVE
ON ONE INCOME?

G oing through breast cancer with Phyllis made me think of my own personal situation. That may sound selfish, but I've always thought a husband and father has to be selectively selfish at times to protect his family. That may mean taking care of his responsibilities with little regard to what others think he should or should not be doing with his time.

I was determined to help ease her concerns in any way possible, and I found there was no room for laziness. Living by my own Rule #1 that it wasn't about me anymore, I chose to take care of myself along with Phyllis. I became more attuned to the dynamics of running a household and that meant making sure we had dinner, taking care of household chores like laundry, and doing my best at keeping a stable income flowing. It's amazing what an individual can accomplish when they are focused.

Two incomes families are the norm in today's society, so many women worry that with a breast cancer diagnosis, the family's financial survival is at risk. Would they lose the house? Would they have to file bankruptcy? I became more motivated than ever to succeed because I knew Phyllis functioned at a higher standard without financial stress. Less stress equals a healthier wife, and worries about money equaled stress for Phyllis.

In April 2013, the year before Phyllis' breast cancer diagnosis, she and her partner, Johanna Shirley, were considering the possibility of going another direction with their real estate company, RE/MAX Premiere Group. Phyllis' Dad, Johnny was in bad health, and she was helping him with his needs. Johanna was soon to be a new mother. I suggested they sell RE/MAX Premiere Group to me. I would take on the company duties and become the qualifying broker, while they both continued to focus on their strong individual real estate careers and their personal lives more. This would allow the company to stay intact, which was what everyone decided we wanted. So I became the owner and broker.

For several months, we rocked on as a ten-agent company, making enough money to pay the bills but not much more than that. In June of 2013, Phyllis' father passed away, and it was particularly hard for her. She hid her sorrow well in public but privately she was devastated. She was a Daddy's girl that was very much like her father, and they loved each other dearly. I considered him my second father and leaned on him after my own father passed away. He was also my friend, and we shared many philosophical conversations.

> *I was inspired by my wife's resilience and positive outlook on the future.*

Phyllis was diagnosed with breast cancer in July 2014. In October of that year, while still taking chemo treatments, we went to the RE/MAX Dixie Region Broker/Owner Summit in Biloxi, Mississippi. While there, I made a commitment to grow the company. I was inspired by my wife's resilience and positive outlook on the future. I wrote down on a yellow legal pad my goal of increasing the number of agents at RE/MAX Premiere Group by adding five new agents in 2015. It is amazing what we can speak into existence. It really is a mindset. The year of 2015, we proudly grew our company with a total of twelve veteran Realtors that chose to join our team! We were both very proud of that accomplishment.

In 2014, Phyllis was the Incoming President of the Tuscaloosa Association of Realtors, representing over four hundred Realtors. Her duties were to schedule guest speakers for each luncheon and to be responsible for introducing them. She earned the respect of many colleagues during her time as Incoming President while having chemotherapy treatments.

As our company grew, we ran out of space at our present office, so I decided to move to a larger facility. I found a site where we could double our office space, and I went to work designing the layout. It was a lot of fun planning and building, and it turned out to be, I feel, one of the nicest real estate offices in town.

Our success during the year after the breast cancer diagnosis was amazing. Phyllis, with her inspiring never-quit attitude, and I ended up as the Alabama RE/MAX Broker of the Year and Alabama RE/MAX Recruiter of the Year. I was surprised with both awards but was honored to receive them. I felt it had been a team effort and was proud that we had made the decision to keep moving forward and looking toward the future while she was in the middle of chemotherapy in 2014.

Now, I said all that to demonstrate that we actually made *more* money the year of Phyllis' breast cancer! I'd resolved to work harder to support my family on one income, if need be. And Phyllis continued selling real estate throughout her surgery and chemotherapy treatments, so in the end we really never had to see if we could live on one income. But since RE/MAX Premiere Group was on my shoulders, that took a tremendous load off her. The company's success created a much-needed energy in our office, which was very important to her.

I pray that you do not think me a braggart because I'm not. God has blessed me and my family immensely, and I am humbled by it and grateful. But I felt it worthy of telling how our finances never suffered but actually flourished as a result of our reliance and interdependence during her battle with breast cancer.

Chapter 20

WILL HE BE FAITHFUL TO YOU?

Breast cancer leaves scars on a woman's body, makes her feel fatigued, and zaps her of vitality for a while. Sometimes the emotional scars are worse than the physical scars. I've known Phyllis for most of her life and this was the lowest point, self-esteem-wise, of her life. She wanted more privacy and would lock her bathroom—she had never done that in the past. She had always been beautiful, and she hated that her chest was missing one breast and that she was bald. She felt ugly, and she was vulnerable. Of course, I let her have her privacy, but she wasn't ugly and that isn't just my biased opinion.

I'd always been very attracted to Phyllis and that was especially

I'd always been very attracted to Phyllis and that was especially true during breast cancer.

true during breast cancer. Through her battle with breast cancer, I learned what true intimacy is. Our marriage had not been perfect by any stretch of the imagination, but through our many disappointments with each other, we had chosen to stick with each other and had not given up. In today's society of lying politicians and celebrity scandals flooding social media, faithfulness and honesty in a marriage is more of an exception to the rule.

After forty-one years of marriage, we finish each other's sentences, she helps me spell, I help her add, she usually makes the bed and I cut the grass, she lets me control the remote, and I stopped complaining about her social media time. I'm looked at in a better light by being married to Phyllis, and I pray the same is true for her being married to me. Over time we figured out our yin and yang. Going through breast cancer with her only solidified my resolve. It made me see things as they really are, and as I've said earlier, one of the hardest things for me was the helpless feeling and not being able to protect her, but I knew I could be faithful to her in many other ways.

I stayed focused, and I worked my tail off with no complaints. All I thought about was how I could make this a little easier on her. I assisted any way I could, whether it be work-related by showing a house for her or going by the pharmacy to get a refill on a prescription or picking up a new one that had been called in. There was always something to do. It sure kept me busy. We went to the Manderson Cancer Center together, and if it had not been for the chemotherapy, I'd say they were the best times we had had together in a very long time.

The Faithful Grizzly

Dr. Hinton had explained to us that while taking chemotherapy, Phyllis' immune system would be weakened. We had many friends and family who came by and visited her, so as her self-appointed gatekeeper, I was worried about them unknowingly sharing some sort of virus with her. I couldn't stop them at the door and make them fill out a questionnaire, so I came up with the idea of putting a friendly reminder at our door.

Visitors who have been in recent contact with any sick or infectious persons . . . please come back at a later date.

Patient's immune system has been weakened by treatments, and we are taking every precaution.

Thank You, Ken

I took some good-natured flak from the family about being over-protective, but I couldn't have cared less. She would have never addressed the issue on her own, and she did not tell me to remove it from the door. So, in a small way, I got to be the protector after all.

I worried about Phyllis' eating habits, especially in the beginning of chemotherapy and every third treatment. Much like her daddy and her bonnet-wearing Grandmother Pearl, I was constantly trying to feed her. I brought home lots of things I thought she might like to eat. I tried tomato soup, which she usually loves, but the acidic flavor hurt the sores in her mouth caused by chemotherapy. Thankfully she was able to drink some homemade Better Boy tomato juice her sister, Becky, brought. She said it reminded her of her Mother and Daddy because they had given it to her when she was sick as a little girl. I generally fought a losing battle that seemed to always end with her wrinkling her nose and shaking her head no with a nauseous expression . . . until I brought home cold watermelon chunks from Publix. That was something she couldn't get enough of, so I kept a plentiful supply.

I never tired of doing for her. I surprised myself in many ways because neither one of us is really good at feeling sorry for the other for a long period of time. We are both tough and expect the other to be tough as well. That's one thing that attracts us to each other. If I'm ever sick, she might pamper me a little, but after a day or two it's like, "Okay, it's time for you to get well!" It might take me three or four days before I'm tired of the sick patient routine! I never felt that way this time, though, and I always looked forward to doing anything I could for her because it was my only way of participating in the process.

Would I be unfaithful to Phyllis? The answer is no. Even with the physical struggles you have with physical intimacy during chemotherapy, being unfaithful was the last thing on my mind. I pray she had no worries regarding this issue because I felt our marriage was stronger than it had ever been.

The physicality of a marriage is important to both men and women, but side effects from chemotherapy can be difficult in this regard. I tried to always keep in mind that the number one thing in life at this time was Phyllis getting well. Nothing else mattered, and this attitude definitely made my marriage stronger and more intimate.

Intimacy doesn't have to be all about the physical. Going through

> *Intimacy doesn't have to be all about the physical.*

this tough period as a couple helped me rediscover the other things that attracted me to Phyllis in the first place. I was keenly aware of the gift of our closeness and the secrets we share. I realized we are still buddies that have each other's backs. She is my best friend.

The big question behind the question is, "Do you still have sex when you're going through breast cancer treatments?" The answer is yes, but you need talk to your doctor about it. Our doctor warned us that we should use protection, especially after a chemotherapy treatment because the drugs can transfer from one partner to the other during intercourse. This could lead to the partner having the same side effects as the patient. Breast cancer treatments have such a profound effect on a woman's body that physical intimacy may be extremely painful. But it may not be an issue for every woman. I learned that love isn't just about physical intimacy. I wanted Phyllis for who she was to me and not for what she could do for me. Those little looks we now shared, reading each other's thoughts and connecting on another level, or when I placed a cool washcloth on her forehead and she whispered her thanks, knowing that I accepted her exactly as she was. That was truly enlightening and brought me all the pleasure I needed.

Chapter 21

RECONSTRUCTION

The notion of "reconstruction" implies something is defective or damaged or misshapen. Imagine how this notion affects a woman who has recently lost one or both breasts. After she has been victimized by breast cancer and has to have a mastectomy, she is now considered by society as defective or damaged! Add that to the fact that society puts way too much emphasis on breasts to begin with.

Of course, this breast infatuation is hardly a new phenomenon. King Solomon, said to be the wisest man who ever lived, wrote about breasts and their beauty. Remember those verses? We read them in church as kids, giggling on the back row! So, what's a woman to do when her breasts are gone? Is she less of a woman? Not in my eyes, but I knew Phyllis felt she wasn't as much a woman as she once was after her mastectomy. And that's not a good place for any woman to be.

At the time of diagnosis, in our initial meeting with Dr. Hinton in July 2014, he informed us of all options for reconstruction. The first option he mentioned was to begin the reconstruction at the time of the mastectomy. This would involve deciding on the plastic surgeon, consulting with him or her about what exactly Phyllis wanted, such as overall breast size. If she chose this route, she would have most likely had expanders placed in her chest immediately at the time of the mastectomy.

So, let that sink in: eleven days prior to this meeting, we were unaware Phyllis even had breast cancer, and now we were imagining a surgical option that included deciding what size replacement breast she wanted.

Another option was to have the mastectomy, let it heal, have chemotherapy, and then have the surgery to put the expanders in. This is called delayed reconstruction.

The next option was to not have reconstructive surgery at all.

As I sat with her and Dr. Hinton, she asked me what I thought. I told her it was her decision and I would support her whichever option she chose, assuring her I was fine with waiting until she had gone through all her treatments. This was what she wanted to do all along. She didn't want to have to make these reconstruction decisions at this particular time and wanted to proceed with caution. This very personal decision worked best for her and is in no way a reflection on others who choose to have reconstructive surgery at the time of the mastectomy. We have friends who chose to combine the surgeries, and it worked fine. It really is a personal decision made by the patient and their physician.

After Phyllis finished her chemotherapy treatments, she began trying to decide if she would even have reconstructive surgery or not. She was feeling like her old self, and the thought of having another surgery was frightening. Finally, she decided she would proceed and began the task of choosing another surgeon for yet another surgery because of this breast cancer journey. I was still helpless but supportive, as was my only choice. And let's face it, I was getting accustomed to the lack of control. Once she made her decision, she became excited with the possibilities of getting a new breast and a chance to feel like a complete woman again! I was beginning to see glimpses of my former confident wife.

On the first day of November 2015, sixteen months after discovering she had breast cancer, Phyllis met with Dr. John Menard the plastic surgeon she had chosen for the reconstructive surgery for a fact-finding meeting. Phyllis didn't need me to hold her hand for this part of the adventure, so she went alone. She had gotten nothing but positive feedback from the many women that were Dr. Menard's patients. I was always amazed at how open most women were when discussing their experiences with Phyllis after having their breasts enhanced and/ or having reconstructive surgery. One lady even displayed the surgeon's handy work to Phyllis. I call that going the extra mile! I wasn't there, but Phyllis said she was a little red-faced. Still, I think she appreciated the gesture.

Dr. Menard was much more than a surgeon. He was more an artist that took his job seriously and strove for perfection. He understood how important his work was to the individual and not only repaired the physical consequences of breast cancer, but he also helped repair their dreams of being normal again. He became our friend.

On November 23, Dr. Menard begin the reconstruction of her breast that had been removed by marking her up. When Phyllis showed me the results of the pre-surgery mark-up meeting, it reminded me of a sad time when she had the mastectomy. The good doctor had drawn on her like a power point presentation graph with lines and arrows. It was his blueprint for success. The next day at DCH Hospital, an expander that was a bladder-like device, would be placed between the interior wall of her chest and underneath the skin. It would be pumped up a little at the time with silicone to allow the skin to stretch slowly to create space for the implant.

The next morning, I took Phyllis to the Same Day Surgery at Tuscaloosa DCH where we ironically parked on the same Level 2 of the parking deck, which is the same level to the entrance to the Manderson Cancer Center. Neither of us looked over that way as we entered the Same Day Surgery entrance. I knew the drill well by now that included pre-op with the nurses and all their paperwork and then waiting on the doctor to arrive to

> . . . *even though she was getting a part of her womanhood back with a breast implant, her empty chest had been her badge of honor.*

perform the surgery. It was somewhat easier saying goodbye that day, I guess because it was an elective surgery, and I felt we were getting a little control back. I watched for her number on the monitor again and knew when she was out of surgery and in recovery. Soon Dr. Menard called for me, and we went into the private room with two chairs and he informed me the surgery went perfectly. I thanked him, and he told me how great Phyllis was. I brought her home that afternoon after she was fully awake with a semblance of a new breast. A small perfectly-shaped mound replaced the empty space on her chest that had a horizontal scar where her old breast had been before the mastectomy. To me it was bittersweet because even though she was getting a part of her womanhood back with a breast implant, her empty chest had been her badge of honor. It was a reminder of what she had overcome and the strength and integrity she had shown. I was happy for her, and I loved her regardless of what her chest looked like.

The expander surgery caused her more pain, but she now no longer needed the prosthetics that filled her bra. That was a welcome change for her. The things women go through to be the best they can be amaze me. I could see her confidence growing again.

After many more follow-ups with physicians that included silicone injections in the expander and deciding whether to go big or not, February 16, 2016, Phyllis finally was able to have the expanders removed and an implant put in its place. It turned out Phyllis needed implants on both sides to, as Dr. Menard stated, "balance her out."

Finally, Phyllis was feeling normal again! She was satisfied with the results of Dr. Menard's work, and her hair had grown back so there was no need for the scarves and wigs anymore. No more worrying at the beach that her wig would blow off in the sea breeze or that the prosthetic would fall out of her bathing suit top.

You would think, "Okay, it's finally over" but no, there's more work to do to satisfy the artist/physician Menard! Remember, Phyllis had her entire breast cut off her body, and that included removing a nipple and areola. So, on September 1, 2016, Phyllis went back to the Tuscaloosa Surgical Center to have a new nipple constructed. The doctor pulled the skin up on her new breast to form a matching nipple. Amazing. After picking out a perfect tattoo color in December, she went to his office for a tattooed areola. She got her tattoo and had a spring in her step like when some random guy whistles at a girl. A girl may scoff at how crude the whistler is, but it seems to always puts a spring in her step!

Two and one-half years after being diagnosed with breast cancer, Phyllis' body was whole again, and it was over. But it is never really over.

Chapter 22

FEAR OF THE FUTURE

Phyllis' body had betrayed her. She had been committed throughout her life to clean living—watching what she ate and exercising consistently. But she had gotten breast cancer in spite of her efforts. It's difficult to trust when you've been betrayed, and such is the case now. Will the cancer come back? Once you have cancer you never really get over the possibility it will return. It's forever in the back of your mind, and how you choose to deal with life after cancer is as important as how you choose to deal with a breast cancer diagnosis. Phyllis and I both are positive individuals, and we go about our lives with faith in God and in ourselves, but breast cancer had hit us with the realization of how fragile life is. That isn't necessarily a bad thing. It will make you better if you let it.

Phyllis' future will always include visits to physicians monitoring her body to make sure the cancer doesn't return or, if it does, to treat it as quickly as possible. Her new normal is visiting the doctors every three-to-six months for blood work and weighing for any sudden weight loss. She still has to have a mammogram of both breasts, and that includes the new breast. They now pull the implant up as far as possible to scan the underside near her chest wall. A MUGA scan will always be in her follow-up treatment because the physician is always looking for a possible return of cancer. DEXA scans and Prolea shots are thrown in for good measure to aid with bone density that may have been affected by previous treatments.

She now has a full body visual scanning to locate and remove any possible moles that could become cancerous. This is her new normal, and she is content with it. She has always been proactive with her health. I kid her that she will go to the doctor when she is well but hates to go when she's sick. I guess she likes good news the best, and who can blame her.

Phyllis fights the urge to eat unhealthy foods but will eat a good hamburger once in a while. She has always taken care of herself, and she tirelessly tries to include me in her regimen. I'm better than I once was, but I'm not radical about it.

> *We try hard to not let breast cancer be what defines Phyllis and internally we do a good job.*

Neither of us lives in constant fear, but only a fool would forget past experiences and not learn from them. We are constantly reminded of breast cancer and there's no getting away from it. Friends, family, and acquaintances are always sharing with us the story of someone they know that is fighting the disease because they know we can relate. I guess it's something we will never get away from, especially from those close to us. We try hard to not let breast cancer be what defines Phyllis and internally we do a good job. Controlling the thoughts of others is impossible when many typically see breast cancer when they see Phyllis.

Living life to the fullest after cancer is truly a faith-based journey. Focusing on breast cancer returning is a losing game. Instead, we hold tight to our faith and that we are in God's hands, and he will take care of us. We look back on his faithfulness and remember Philippians 4:4: "Rejoice in the Lord always. I will say it again, Rejoice!"

Philippians 4:4: "Rejoice in the Lord always. I will say it again, Rejoice!"

Chapter 23

FROM THE HEART

Although I tried to be positive throughout the diagnosis, treatments, and the reconstructive surgery, it was a very arduous time in my life. Time moved slowly, and I must admit I wished the time away on several occasions, wanting the treatments and everything about breast cancer to be over so we could get back to our normal life. But then I asked myself, "What did I want to get back to?" It wasn't so much I loved my old routine—I just wanted to be able to stop worrying about Phyllis' health. I never felt sorry for myself, but I did feel for her.

This thing changed my life. I was in a rut of dealing with real estate issues and managing Realtors, reading emails, and then coming home and maybe cooking a little supper and getting in my recliner to flip the channels and my life away. Sad, when you think about it. A few times in my life I've made the statement to Phyllis that I need to shake things up and chose a new path to go down. Breast cancer did the shaking up this time, and I didn't like it.

> *The only way to become relevant was to become a humble servant.*

When I first found out that Phyllis had breast cancer on July 18, 2014, I was flooded with a bevy of emotions from disbelief to anger. But I had nowhere to direct my anger, and who was I to be angry with any of this? I really didn't matter in this deal, and my self-imposed Rule #1 was that it's not about me. The only way to become relevant was to become a humble servant. I've always had a servant's heart, but my humility has been a struggle for me at times.

I wondered why they—whomever *they* are—couldn't find a cure for breast cancer. I considered if they did find a cure, would they let the public quickly know about it, or would it take decades to be approved? It's a billion dollar-a-year business, and they won't let that go easily. All these thoughts trickled into my head when I was feeling impotent in my ability to control the situation. I did my best at hiding these

> *Whenever I think of the times my children wondered if their mother was dying and how they tried to be strong through it all—well, it's about more than I can bear.*

thoughts and feelings and never shared them with anyone until now. Being strong is always a tough job if you rely on yourself. I had to rely on a faith in God I'd nearly forgotten I had.

It's funny—sometimes now I can be a blubbering idiot, tearing up at the least of things. Like George W. Bush who wouldn't make eye contact with his dad during his own inauguration because, as he said, "we're a family of weepers." I cry easily these days. This book project has prompted many tears. I've had to revisit trying times that I had no control over. Whenever I think of the times my children wondered if their mother was dying and how they tried to be strong through it all—well, it's about more than I can bear. I barely wrote that last sentence without breaking down! When I remember Phyllis and Caroline holding each other in bed, crying and praying after first finding out the diagnosis and at that moment Phyllis deciding she must be strong for her kids, I become an emotional wreck. When I was growing up, all my friends and I wanted to be tough guys, and we knew no tough guys that cried. Until this journey, I shed very few tears unless my family was hurting, but I learned through this that it's okay to cry. When I think of the outpouring of sentiment from friends and folks we didn't really know, I'm deeply touched. That letter from our young neighbor, Quinn Edmonds, encouraging "Mrs. Phyllis," moves me in ways I've never experienced. Even at his young age he knew the physical and emotional pain cancer causes.

With my newfound ability to cry at the drop of a hat, I've learned something new, and that is that it takes strength to be open in front of your loved ones. It really doesn't mean I'm less of anything, and it sure makes me more human. Maybe it's part of the aging process. I remember my Dad becoming that way in his later years, and if crying is a part of getting old, then I'm beginning to accept and like the old me.

I discovered a peace that can only come from trusting in a higher power to lead me through a time of powerlessness.

It seems almost sacrilegious to say this, but breast cancer made Phyllis and me better people. Better together and better individually. We found ways to work together better. It forced me to put her needs above my own. I discovered a peace that can only come from trusting in a higher power to lead me through a time of powerlessness. I was reminded that God is in control, and He will not put more on us than we can bear.

I do not think for one minute that God puts cancer on anyone. I think God wants us to live a productive and happy life with a servant's heart. As Phyllis went about her duties, she didn't use her problems as an excuse. I was proud as she continued as Incoming President of the Tuscaloosa Association of Realtors through the weekly chemotherapy, and even after those treatments were over, although weakened, she persevered as President the next year while taking Herceptin every third week. Standing in front of her colleagues each month took courage, and I don't know that I could have done that. I could only support her with my attendance at the meetings because I knew it was important to her.

I pray we never have to deal with any type of cancer again and that we both live long disease-free lives. I pray a cure will be found for all cancers. I do believe God still heals, and I believe he healed Phyllis and we both realize we were blessed with good results. Every cancer story doesn't have a good ending. Four of Phyllis' friends taking chemotherapy treatments while she did, lost their battle. All fought valiantly but passed on. We still miss fellow Realtor Debbie Merrill, friend David Reynolds, childhood friend Eddie Alexander and buddy Jimmy Kuykendall.

I guess the highest compliment I can pay Phyllis is that I think of her as a Proverbs 31 woman. Several of those memorable verses stand out to me. Verse 11, her husband trusts her. Verse 16, she looks at land, buys it, and then plants a vineyard on it. Verse 20, she gives to those in need. Verse 28, her husband and children respect her. Verse 29 is my favorite: "She's the best." Proverbs 31 describes my wife Phyllis and that suits me to a "T". Being the quiet leader she is, she inspires others by living a victorious life, steadfastly refusing to be a victim.

Phyllis has said she's glad her Dad didn't have to see her go through breast cancer because it would have hurt him so, but I know he would have been proud of her and would have tried to feed her back to health with fresh tomato juice. I'm proud that I got to be the one to feed her watermelon and hold her hand. And I pray the Lord gives me many more years to hold that hand and be her loving husband.

Acknowledgments

Thank you to my agent, Bruce Barbour, for leading me in the right direction for publishing this book. Additional thanks to my editor, Ami McConnell, for her patience with a rookie writer with big dreams. I discovered the bittersweet writing process of putting myself back in a difficult time with the hope of maybe bringing a small peace to a few.

I'm also grateful to Morgan James Publishing and their professional team for seeing what I saw in this account of my family's journey through breast cancer. And to Karli Jackson for cleaning it all up.

United States Breast Cancer Statistics

- About 1 in 8 U.S. women (about 12%) will develop invasive breast cancer over the course of her lifetime.
- In 2017, an estimated 252,710 new cases of invasive breast cancer are expected to be diagnosed in women in the U.S., along with 63,410 new cases of non-invasive (in situ) breast cancer.
- About 2,470 new cases of invasive breast cancer are expected to be diagnosed in men in 2017. A man's lifetime risk of breast cancer is about 1 in 1,000.
- Breast cancer incidence rates in the U.S. began decreasing in the year 2000, after increasing for the previous two decades. They dropped by 7% from 2002 to 2003 alone. One theory is that this decrease was partially due to the reduced use of hormone replacement therapy (HRT) by women after the results of a large study called the Women's Health Initiative were published in 2002. These results suggested a connection between HRT and increased breast cancer risk.
- About 40,610 women in the U.S. are expected to die in 2017 from breast cancer, though death rates have been decreasing since 1989. Women under 50 have experienced larger decreases.

These decreases are thought to be the result of treatment advances, earlier detection through screening, and increased awareness.

- For women in the U.S., breast cancer death rates are higher than those for any other cancer, besides lung cancer.

- Besides skin cancer, breast cancer is the most commonly diagnosed cancer among American women. In 2017, it's estimated that about 30% of newly diagnosed cancers in women will be breast cancers.

- In women under 45, breast cancer is more common in African-American women than white women. Overall, African-American women are more likely to die of breast cancer. For Asian, Hispanic, and Native-American women, the risk of developing and dying from breast cancer is lower.

- As of March 2017, there are more than 3.1 million women with a history of breast cancer in the U.S. This includes women currently being treated and women who have finished treatment.

- About 5-10% of breast cancers can be linked to gene mutations (abnormal changes) inherited from one's mother or father. Mutations of the BRCA1 and BRCA2 genes are the most common. On average, women with a BRCA1 mutation have a 55-65% lifetime risk of developing breast cancer. For women with a BRCA2 mutation, the risk is 45%. Breast cancer that is positive for the BRCA1 or BRCA2 mutations tends to develop more often in younger women. An increased ovarian cancer risk is also associated with these genetic mutations. In men, BRCA2 mutations are associated with a lifetime breast cancer risk of about 6.8%; BRCA1 mutations are a less frequent cause of breast cancer in men.

- About 85% of breast cancers occur in women who have no family history of breast cancer. These occur due to genetic mutations that happen as a result of the aging process and life in general, rather than inherited mutations.

- The most significant risk factors for breast cancer are gender (being a woman) and age (growing older).

Information found on breastcancer.org[2]

Just for the Men

- We may never know why we go through certain events in our lives. Maybe it's so our future generations will benefit. Hopefully they can benefit from our mistakes.
- I came to terms with parts of our relationship that needed letting go of. I chose to not let them matter anymore. I decided to forgive and ask for forgiveness.
- You will not ignore cancer. It is so painful to consider a loved one having this dreaded disease, but there is hope. Great strides have been made in the fight against breast cancer.
- Men, try to keep things as normal as possible. Breast cancer will eventually become part of your new normal, but meanwhile you need to display stability. This is critical because most everyone else will be looking at her and wondering if she is dying. When they see her, they will see breast cancer, and there's nothing you can do about that.
- You might as well join the breast cancer club. This club consists of women who have had breast cancer or have a close connection with a loved one who has experienced it. They all have a unique story to tell, and women are verbal by nature, so enjoy it. You can be a silent observer and learn a little about how women operate.

- You will be judged by how you treat your partner. Especially by women. If you lift her up and support her, you will be viewed as a champion.
- Taking time out to be with her during treatments is the best way to show you care.
- Go with her every time you can to her appointments. Be attentive while the physician is talking. This is important to you and her. You'll become part of the process and know what to expect. She will love you for it.
- Take her lunch or breakfast while she is at chemotherapy.
- Take enough for the nursing staff.
- Buy the most expensive gifts you can for her. She deserves it. It will let her know you still care about her and think of her as your friend and lover.
- Take care of the bills. I know you can add and subtract. It's as simple as buying a new gun to hunt with or fishing gear to go fishing with.
- Give her space when she wants it. If you're under her feet constantly she may think you think she's not going to make it.
- Find a routine that works for you and her. We all love habits.
- Get her out of the house. She can sit in the passenger side of a car as easy as she can rest in a recliner. The fresh air will do you both good.
- She may become adventurous and suddenly want to experience a more exciting life. Hang on and enjoy.
- She may become more spiritual. Remember she has come face-to-face with the reality of death. Try praying together and pray for someone besides yourself.
- There will be a few that don't care she has breast cancer, and there may be some that are a little happy about it. This reality may be hard to accept, but it's true. Pray for them too.

- She's going to look different, so deal with it.
- Make lemonade out of life's lemons.
- Circumstances do not create character. They *reveal* character.
- Take care of yourself. She's not your momma.
- Seek help if you need it. Church is a good place to find it. Christians want to help you.
- Keep a journal with her throughout this journey. I regretfully admit I did not.
- Love her like there's no tomorrow!

About the Author

Ken resides in Tuscaloosa, Alabama, with his wife Phyllis. They own RE/MAX Premiere Group real estate company where Ken is the qualifying broker and Phyllis continues listing and selling homes. Ken enjoys his work and family. Especially Olivia and Marlys, his lovely granddaughters.

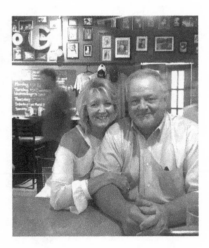

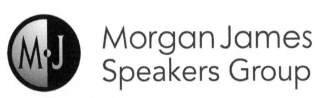

Morgan James
Speakers Group

⏵ www.TheMorganJamesSpeakersGroup.com

We connect Morgan James published
authors with live and online events
and audiences who will benefit
from their expertise.

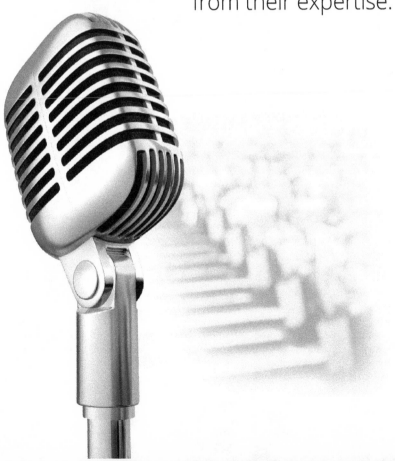

CPSIA information can be obtained
at www.ICGtesting.com
Printed in the USA
BVHW08s1818020918
526305BV00002B/223/P